Preface

The unique recipe of mixing the art and science of medicine with the needs of the insurance and legal community is what makes the provision of a quality independent medical evaluation so difficult.

Interestingly, if you utter the words "IME" to medical students, residents, or fellows, you probably will get a blank stare. These evaluations are typically not on the radar screen within formal medical education curricula, and the common physician does not hear about them until they are well into establishing their own practices.

But this fact is often lost upon those who rely upon these evaluations to establish certain medical opinions within the context of a claim and those who seek out experts who are able to effectively communicate this information.

Thus, there has yet to be formalized a standard textbook or universal educational program that not only teaches the basics of IME provision but also can serve as a reference manual for those who already perform such services.

This book is written to achieve those goals. It is intended to define the IME product and provide information on how to establish these professional services. The text includes essential information for physicians in a "how-to" format, using example templates. Common challenges and pitfalls are discussed, with strategies and pearls shared to illustrate how to avoid them.

Sioux City, Iowa, USA — Douglas W. Martin, MD

Acknowledgments

There are so many people that I would like to thank that I am sure I am going to leave someone out, so my apologies if I have missed someone.

First to my wife, Janet, who has stood by me and raised our four children while tutoring our Haitian son, Caleb, as he fulfills his native country's need for health-care workers. She has "put up" with my challenges as an occupational medicine physician and my genetic love of teaching that frequently requires me to be away from home.

To my children, Kendall, Kylie, Kaleb, and Kaden, who remind me why I get up and go to work each day.

To my parents, Jerry and Kay Martin. Both are educators, my father, who we lost in 2011 (I will carry his dedication and worldly perspective forever), and my mother, still going strong 10 years post liver transplant, whose love is enduring.

To those teachers and coaches way back in high school who instilled in me "this is the way it's done and why": Fred and Marianne Applegate, Arlen Schroeder, Mary and Betty Heard, Dave Bell, Mike Krambeck, Mike Harris, George Snodgrass, Rogers Smith, Don Tietjen, Robert Grigg, Iro Johnson, and Jim Doty.

To my brothers in Beta Sigma Psi at the University of Nebraska–Lincoln. Per aspera ad astra.

To my mentors in medical education: LeeRoy Meyer, MD, at UNMC, and Drs. Monte Skaufle and Dean Bunting in Davenport, Iowa.

To my friends and colleagues in the American Academy of Disability Evaluating Physicians/International Academy of Independent Medical Evaluators (AADEP/IAIME) whom I have relied on constantly: Mark Pilley, Bill Blair, Randy Lea, Phil Osborne, Marc Taylor, Russell Travis, Bob Barth, Ed Klimek, Ron Zipper, Mark Melhorn, and especially Jim Talmage who reads the medical literature with the fervor of a hawk.

To my friends and colleagues at the Iowa Academy of Family Physicians (IAFP) including former executive Janet Wee who nudged me into the world of service to physician organizations.

To my friends and colleagues at the American College of Occupational and Environmental Medicine (ACOEM) who have always had my back no matter what, especially Merris Young, Jim Butler, Dave McKinney, Rich Johnson, and Scott Spillmann.

To everyone at UnityPoint Health Occupational Medicine in Sioux City who allowed me to "do what I do" and do it in a manner that I am proud of.

Contents

About the Author

Douglas W. Martin, MD is an occupational medicine physician who practices in Sioux City, Iowa. Originally trained as a family physician, he has conducted over a thousand medicolegal evaluations in his 23-year career. In addition to examinations related to workers' compensation claims on both state and federal levels, he performs independent medical evaluations for personal injury claimants and defendants, the Social Security System, and disability insurance carriers. Using his training in family medicine, he brings a unique perspective to the concepts of biopsychosocial implications of injury recovery as well as claim behavior.

Dr. Martin is a past president of the International Academy of Independent Medical Evaluators (formerly known as the American Academy of Disability Evaluating Physicians), the Iowa Academy of Family Physicians, and the Iowa Academy of Family Physicians Foundation. He is the founder and a past president of Veritas Medicus, the AADEP Foundation, and was lead author and editor of the book *CRPS – What is the Evidence?*, a volunteer effort of that organization.

He has taught at over 400 continuing medical education events and is a primary educator for the American College of Occupational and Environmental Medicine, chairing its Musculoskeletal Examination and Treatment Techniques core curriculum course and AMA Guides to the Evaluation of Permanent Impairment course. He has taught foundational principles of IME provision and application of the AMA Guides to the Evaluation of Permanent Impairment for over 20 years to ACOEM as well as to IAIME (AADEP) course attendees. In 2015, he was presented with AADEP's first Lifetime Achievement Award for his years of service as officer, educator, author, AMA House of Delegates Representative, CME guru, certification examination committee chair, charity auctioneer, and Jeopardy competition emcee.

He is heavily involved in the leadership roles in organized medicine, serving as Medical Review Officer Section Chair and Private Practice Section Secretary-Treasurer for ACOEM, as well as Speaker of their House of Delegates. He is a 10-year member of the AMA House of Delegates and a 4-year member of the AAFP Congress of Delegates.

His nonmedical time is spent in many charitable endeavors. First and foremost, he is a 35-year veteran of scouting and is both an Eagle Scout and Silver Beaver. Dr. Martin is a founding member of the Tri State Youth Association (www.tristateyouthsd.org) and is heavily involved in supporting Haiti missions via an organization that his wife, Janet, cofounded, Time4Haiti (www.Time4Haiti.org).

Dr. Martin grew up in Louisville, Nebraska, a small town of 1000 people on the Platte River, and is a product of the University of Nebraska educational system graduating with a BS in Biological Sciences from the Lincoln campus and an MD from UNMC in Omaha. He lives in Dakota Dunes, South Dakota, and has four children. When he has spare time, he enjoys Canadian coin collecting and following the University of Nebraska Cornhuskers.

1 What Is an Independent Medical Evaluator?

An independent medical evaluator is usually a physician who performs a healthcare evaluative service as a third party at the request of an advocate who is involved in a medicolegal claim. The phrase "independent medical examination" is also sometimes used. However, for obvious reasons, it reflects a narrower scope of practice in that an actual examination of an individual claimant occurs. It is preferred, therefore, to use the phrase "independent medical evaluation" as this would also encompass activities, such as file reviews, where a physical examination does not take place.

These services are usually requested by employers or insurance carriers within the workers' compensation benefit system but are also commonly performed in legal cases where there has been a claim of injury or illness caused by one party upon another.

Within our US legal system, decision-makers such as judges, juries, and commissions, commonly referred to as "triers of fact," are responsible for determining whether an injury has occurred that is compensable by some form of monetary award. Thus, the independent medical evaluator is often looked upon to offer a professional opinion as to not only whether an injury or illness has actually occurred, but whether it is a temporary or permanent issue. In the case of a permanent medical problem, it is necessary within the claim process to determine the severity and extent of the medical issue, so that a reasonable monetary award can be decided to compensate the injured party.

There are other reasons that an independent medical evaluation (IME) might be requested. Within the workers compensation benefit system, an injured party may be undergoing medical treatment that the employer or employer's insurance carrier is questioning. Often, IMEs are requested in this situation when the treating physician has requested advanced diagnostic testing, or where a treatment, such as a surgery is of high cost. Given that the costs of care within the workers compensation system are higher for the same medical diagnoses compared to the general medical population, these IMEs are often directed due to a concern of cost/benefit analysis insofar as the question arises as to whether a test or treatment is necessary to

D.W. Martin, *Independent Medical Evaluation*,
https://doi.org/10.1007/978-3-319-71906-1_1

effectuate a good outcome, which is almost always measured in terms of successful return to work.

There may be also legitimate reasons for an employer or insurance carrier to request an IME when there is "delayed recovery"; meaning a situation where the injured worker is not at a point of healing or return to work compared to expected normative time frames. Given that there are many reasons for recovery delays in workers compensation claims, the IME physician is often asked to determine whether these issues are related to the severity of the medical problem, or some other outside factor frequently referred to as "psycho-social-economic" incentives.

It is known that in the workers compensation context, a worker's treating physician may be, sometimes, unknowingly contributing to the prolonged recovery due to a misplaced sense of patient advocacy. Additionally, where there are interpersonal conflicts with an employment arrangement or a deconditioned individual who struggles with a job task where the issue is intolerance of an activity as opposed to injury, there is a tendency to inappropriately medically legitimize excessive and extended treatments. Thus, the IME provider can shed some light on these issues as an impartial opinion is often more objective than what the treating provider can offer.

While less common, IMEs may be requested in long-term disability (LTD) claims. Usually, the issue arises out of an LTD claim that has been submitted by a covered person to an insurance carrier. LTD insurance is quite common in the United States and is often offered as an employment benefit to workers. When illness or catastrophic injuries occur that prevent the individual from returning to work, LTD policies provide some residual level of income typically for the remainder of the person's work life.

In reviewing LTD claims, insurance carriers will rely heavily upon the medical records submitted by the claimants treating physicians. And, it is the norm that these records are able to provide enough information for the claim reviewer to make a determination as to whether the medical issues raise to the level where the LTD policy terms would apply. However, there are some instances where either the medical condition is not clear or is controversial where the medical records do not allow an easy coverage determination. Also, there are situations where they may be questions of severity of functional limitation for a given medical condition and also whether the level of functional limitation is permanent, can be mitigated to allow successful return to work, or accommodated in other ways by an employer. In these situations, an IME can be requested to address any or all of these questions.

On the other hand, personal injury lawsuits are common in the United States. The IME physician can play an important role in providing an unbiased opinion regarding the extent of a claimed injury as well as the impact that the injury may have on future earnings capacity. Frequently, the litigants within a personal injury case will be especially focused upon the level of "pain and suffering" since monetary damages can be awarded within these types of lawsuits and not in others. As a physician, the IME provider can also communicate opinions regarding future care needs and the impact of pain upon function, which are often lynchpins of determining the amount of monetary awards given in these claims.

Obviously, it is important for the IME physician to understand the motivation of the claimants within a personal injury lawsuit. It is commonplace for evaluators to witness anger, skepticism, and a variety of other negative emotions as part of this process. Although these emotions can be a part of all litigated medical claims, they seem to be heightened within these types of lawsuits, as they typically involve higher dollar demands. Also as important is to understand the impact that these emotions can play not only in a mental health context but also when mental health problems manifest themselves into actual physical maladies, frequently referred to as "somatization."

Another note regarding personal injury lawsuits is to recognize the number of these claims that arise from motor vehicle accidents. Given the sheer number of automobiles and accident rates in the United States, the IME physician should be prepared that a great number of evaluations requested will originate from these events. Thus, the physician should be experienced to the level that they understand, at least to a reasonable level, human ergonomics and mechanisms of injury that exist within typical car crashes. To that end, dedicated consulting companies exist that focus only on these issues, and the IME provider may find it helpful to explore additional training and education in this area.

While on the subject of training and education, it must be understood by all stakeholders that there is no formal training on the proper provision of an independent medical evaluation in either medical schools or residency programs. The nonmedical stakeholder may be surprised at this; however the traditions and standard practices of the Accreditation Council on Graduate Medical Education (ACGME) and the American Board of Medical Specialties (ABMS) do not contain recommendations on IMEs within their regulations, and no ABMS specialty board certification organization (e.g., the American Board of Family Medicine, the American Board of Preventive Medicine, American Board of Physical Medicine and Rehabilitation) contains a requirement or even a suggestion that IME parameters be taught.

Thus, there is a dichotomy in that the legal needs of having an independent medical evaluation do not mesh with the nonexistent importance paid to it within the formal medical education process. As a result, physicians typically find themselves learning about the very existence of IMEs once they have already established a practice, and then only by indirect means. Some physicians are fortunate to join practices where a colleague or partner is performing this service, and in those situations, a mentoring process occurs. Other physicians may receive inquiries from attorneys or insurance carriers regarding whether they would be willing to provide IME services but may have no idea what the specifics entail.

More commonly, IME services provide an attractive practice alternative to physicians who are looking to change their scope of what they do. Commonly, orthopedic surgeons look to begin performing IMEs later in their careers as a way to segue from being in the operating room and on call to a more scheduled and controlled environment. Some physicians look to IME services as a way to stay involved in the medical field because otherwise they may have a physical impairment that no longer allows them to conduct procedures or other activities. There are also physicians who decide to add IMEs to their service line because it provides them a more consistent revenue stream, unencumbered by negotiated fee discounts, contractual fee adjustments, insurance down-coding, and collection problems that are quite common challenges within usual physician practices. Still others become involved in IME provision because they see it as an integral part of their practice, as is often the case in occupational medicine where involvement within the workers compensation system is frequent, or because they enjoy the intricacies of the medicolegal interface and believe that their scientific and medical roles are important to bring toward often complex issues.

So what options do physicians have who desire education and training in the IME field?

There are, fortunately, a variety of entities that provide continuing medical education (CME) courses on the subject. The currently available organizations that provide these educational opportunities are as follows:

International Academy of Independent Medical Evaluators	www.iaime.org
American Board of Independent Medical Examiners	www.abime.org
American College of Occupational and Environmental Medicine	www.acoem.org
SEAK	www.seak.com

The International Academy of Independent Medical Evaluators (IAIME) was for its first 28 years of existence, known as the American Academy of Disability Evaluating Physicians (AADEP). The name was changed in 2016 to reflect a perspective that's it members provided a variety of IME services that were not solely focused upon disability evaluation. IAIME is primarily focused upon CME provision, offering a variety of courses throughout the year, including a comprehensive training course that is the foundational course of the organization and reflects its beliefs of what should be considered the standard core curriculum for IME physicians.

IAIME is a Specialty Service Society and House of Delegates member of the American Medical Association. Although not an ABMS specialty, IAIME has plans to provide a board certification, expanding upon its prior certificate level credential referred to as CEDIR (Certified Evaluator of Disability and Impairment Rating). The organization does also bestow fellowship, a designation that allows one to become a voting member of the organization and is granted by the accumulation of a certain number of points that can be obtained by completing a variety of different activities.

The American Board of Independent Medical Examiners (ABIME) was originally an organization that was solely focused on certification of IME providers, the first certifications being issued in 1995. Since that time, ABIME has expanded into CME and now also provides a variety of courses that are focused on the AMA impairment rating guides and other medicolegal topics. ABIME is also not an ABMS specialty but does offer a board certification examination, leading to the designation CIME (certified independent medical examiner). They also provide an alternative examination for chiropractors, leading to the designation CICE (certified independent chiropractic examiner).

The American College of Occupational and Environmental Medicine (ACOEM) is also a Specialty Service Society and AMA House of Delegates member and represents approximately 4000 physician members. Although ACOEM does not have a formal dedicated continuing medical education program devoted to IME training, it does provide courses in the AMA Guides to the Evaluation of Permanent Impairment and also traditionally incorporates educational offerings regarding IME provision at its annual meeting, the American Occupational Health Conference. ACOEM provides optional membership in sections, which are entities within the organization where members who have particular interests can share information and dialogue and host their own educational activities. One such section is the Work Fitness and Disability Section, which typically includes ACOEM members who provide IME services within the workers compensation system.

SEAK is a private organization that is a continuing education, publishing, and consulting company. They provide training opportunities for both physicians and non-physicians in the areas of expert witnesses, causation analysis, nonclinical careers, and supplemental income. They publish professional directories for expert witnesses, IME doctors, and file review consultants and have also published several reference texts. They have sponsored an annual worker's compensation and occupational medicine conference since 1980.

Bibliography

1. Demeter S, Andersson G. Disability Evaluation. 2nd ed. St. Louis: Mosby; 2003.
2. Nierenberg C, Brigham C, Direnfield L, Burket C. Standards for Independent Medical Examinations. Guides Newsletter; 2005 Nov/Dec.
3. Rondinelli R, Katz T. Impairment rating and disability evaluation. Philadelphia: Saunders; 2000.
4. American Board of Independent Medical Examiners. www.abime.org. Accessed 25 Sep 2017.
5. American College of Occupational and Environmental Medicine. www.acoem.org. Accessed 25 Sep 2017.
6. International Academy of Independent Medical Evaluators. www.iaime.org. Accessed 25 Sep 2017.
7. SEAK, Inc. www.seak.com. Accessed 25 Sep 2017.

Medicolegal Systems and the IME Provider

2

The purpose of having an independent medical evaluation performed within any medicolegal context is to have on record, a professional medical report which serves as an expert opinion that one side or the other can use to advocate for their argument or claim. Within these contexts, the more definitive the opinion is, the more weight and value it has to the side who is attempting to prove an argument or claim. However, it is imperative to note that the IME opinion must be expressed within the limits of medical knowledge, and since medicine is both art and science, there are often areas where consensus does not exist. This explains why, for example, medical opinions can differ from one IME provider to another.

An IME report may be a requirement of a court or other trier of fact when litigation is pending, or attorneys may want a written report to assist in settlement negotiations prior to hearings or trials. As such, it is critically important that the IME physician understand the context within which the claim lies, as there may be certain jurisdictional rules that dictate not only what sort of evaluation is to occur, but also what sort of information is important to communicate that is then used to satisfy the questions that the disability system requires.

When contemplating the position and purpose of IMEs, frequently the issue of ethics comes into play. From the physician perspective, it is often of considerable debate as to how the role of patient advocacy can influence decision-making especially in terms of disability certification. The true and traditional role of a patient advocate is to always do what is in the best interest of the patient. But a more contemporary view that is practiced by many physicians is to always do what the patient wants. The problem with these two views is that in areas of disability determination, they can be at odds with each other.

When there is a dispute regarding these issues that surround the treating physician's viewpoint, it becomes critical that the IME physician remain impartial. However, many argue that an IME provider can never really be impartial given that they fully know well where the fees for their services are coming from. It is hard for any service industry provider, whether it is medical or otherwise, to set aside issues

D.W. Martin, *Independent Medical Evaluation*,
https://doi.org/10.1007/978-3-319-71906-1_2

of customer satisfaction when payment for a function has a certain expected outcome.

This is a fact not lost upon the courts and judges. Many judges refuse to allow the characterization of these evaluations as "independent" and instead rule that they must be referred to as "defense medical evaluations" or "plaintiff medical evaluations," making a point that it is the counselor or who they represent who are paying the bill for these services, and not the court itself who has directed them to occur. Having said that, there are a few instances, mainly in the individual state worker's compensation programs, where an IME can indeed be requested by the court, but for which the payment for the IME is the responsibility of one side or the other, or in some cases, shared.

Regardless, the prudent IME physician should exercise caution and avoid being stereotyped as "defense" or "plaintiff" friendly. Unfortunately, many stakeholders in medicolegal systems can readily identify IME physician outliers whose opinion can be counted on, despite the specifics of an individual case. These physicians, unfortunately, have tainted to a certain degree, the public's perception of IME providers, and have created phraseology that is unbecoming to doctors of medicine. Such statements and phrases as "his opinion is bought and paid for," "he wouldn't find anything wrong even if I was dead," "the disabling doctor," and "defense whore" echo in the halls of insurance companies and attorney offices across the country.

As such, there is clearly a place for the physician performing IMEs who is willing to make objective and fair determinations. When the IME physician uses sound medical judgment, is comprehensive in their assessment of a medical problem, and applies consistently evidence based decision making, there is little reason to be concerned about the validity and acceptance of their opinions.

A brief review of the various United States disability benefit systems is given in the following sections. These descriptions are not intended to be comprehensive, and there is a focus upon what areas IME physicians are most often asked to address.

State Worker's Compensation Programs

Each state and territory within the United States has its own specific workers' compensation statutes. These laws are intended to establish and administer a no-fault system whereby employees generally forfeit their right to sue their employers and employers give up their immunity that would normally exist in situations where they would not be at fault for an injury or illness.

There are three main benefits that are administered within state workers' compensation programs: survivor benefits in cases of death, medical expense coverage, and wage loss replacement.

Typically, IME physicians are asked in the context of workers' compensation claims to opine on a variety of issues. Since what type of injury or illness is covered under the statutes is defined somewhat differently among the different states, issues of causation and compensability predominate. What medical conditions arise out of the course of employment and are "work-related" are what might be on the surface easy questions to answer but in reality are not especially given the multifactorial origins of many diagnoses. But, they are critically important to answer so that an employee's medical expenses can be assigned to the correct systems that are available. Thus, IME physicians are frequently called upon to offer opinions on medical causation.

Causation analysis is a discipline within medicine that is poorly understood and poorly performed. The reason for this is that, yet again, little training is afforded the physician on the topic in medical school and residency. Also, there is often a false presumption of causation that is based solely upon the chronological presentation of an event and a medical problem; a work-related event occurred, and then a medical problem ensued. Thus, the medical problem *must* be caused by the work related event. This error in judgement is referred to eloquently as *post hoc ergo propter hoc* and is a well-known scientific fallacy.

IME physicians are also often involved when there are issues of delayed recovery, meaning that an injured worker has not recovered and/or not returned to work as expected. There may be many reasons for this: inaccurate diagnosis, inappropriate or ineffective treatment, comorbid conditions, psycho-social-economic drivers, etc. The IME is requested in order to identify these barriers and also to then address them so as to effectuate an improved final outcome.

Other issues that IMEs may address within state workers' compensation systems include determinations of work ability after an injury or illness has been treated, frequently cached in terms of whether or not and individual requires "permanent restrictions." Usually these questions come about because there is a medical problem that has not recovered completely despite optimum treatment. In these situations, it is incumbent upon some physician to declare that the employee has reached "MMI" (maximum medical improvement), a term that has important and significant meaning in state workers' compensation systems that usually trigger the conclusion of medical care but the start of formal final employability determinations as well as impairment determinations.

Lastly, the IME physician will frequently be asked to perform an impairment rating. An impairment rating examination takes place because an injury or illness has caused a loss or loss of use of a body organ or system function, and typically state workers' compensation statutes have a mechanism to compensate the injured worker because of how the medical problem usually translates into a permanent partial disability.

A note of caution is important here in that physicians (and others) will often use the terms "impairment" and "disability" interchangeably, when they in actuality represent two very different concepts. "Impairment" refers to what is permanently wrong with the person. This could be an amputated body part, a limitation in a joint range of motion, or a decrease in pulmonary function. Impairments are usually easily measurable or at least quantifiable by physicians. "Disability" on the other hand, refers to how the impairment translates into how a particular task is performed. Within workers' compensation IMEs, the physician is usually asked to focus on impairment, as most state programs use the concept of an impairment rating as a basis for calculating compensation payments. There are, however, some states that incorporate adjustment factors into this calculation, taking into consideration issues that are more oriented toward disability, such as age, educational level, local employment options, etc.

The "impairment rating" is thus frequently within the purview of the IME physician. Many states use an authoritative guide that the physician uses in order to calculate the rating. Several states use the *AMA Guides to the Evaluation of Permanent Impairment*. There is currently a rather interesting scenario in the United States where different state workers' compensation systems use different editions of the *AMA Guides*, not necessarily the most recent. This has led to widespread philosophical discussion among stakeholders in the workers' compensation systems, but the decision of what edition of the *AMA Guides* to use has been based mainly upon what each state deems most appropriate to strike a balance between worker and employer perspectives. Lastly, there are some states that have published their own impairment rating guides, some of which is based upon portions of the AMA Guides, and some of which are quite individualized.

It is not the purpose of this text to delve into the education and experience necessary to utilize the AMA and state impairment guides correctly. Various different educational offerings and training programs exist that there are a variety of ancillary textbooks and publications that can be helpful. But, know that becoming fluent in the *AMA Guides* is not an easy thing to master, again because of the fact that there is no training provided within the confines of the formal medical educational process.

Federal Workers' Compensation Programs

There are several federal workers' compensation programs, including FECA (Federal Employee's Compensation Act), LHWCA (Longshore and Harbor Workers' Compensation Act), the Federal Black Lung Program, and EEOICPA (Energy Employees Occupational Illness Compensation Program Act). These programs all are administered by the Office of Workers' Compensation Programs which is a division of the US Department of Labor.

FECA acts similar to the individual state workers' compensation systems but covers federal civilian employees including the Postal Service, Peace Corps, and the Federal Air Patrol. It provides for medical care coverage, lost wage benefits, and survivor benefits. Traditionally, FECA claims are less contentious, and the claims' process is dependent more upon quality written reports by the treating physician. However, IMEs are needed when there are concerns about the extent of impairment or when the details of a medical issue cannot be resolved. An interesting fact is that under the federal statutes, compensation awards are not given for spinal injuries unless there is a permanent extremity radiculopathy.

LHWCA also has features similar to FECA with regard to benefit coverage and is intended to cover those workers who are employed in activities on or adjacent to the navigable waters of the United States. Usually, there is little need for causation analysis in these claims because once a claim is made, unless there is some obvious deception, it is usually accepted. The need arises for IMEs in this system mainly when there is a need for an impairment rating as the program uses the *AMA Guides*.

The Federal Black Lung Program was created to provide income protection and medical coverage for miners who are disabled because of pneumoconiosis. Benefits are only awarded if the miner is shown to be completely disabled based upon established criteria set by the Department of Labor regarding chest x-ray findings, pulmonary function tests, and arterial blood gases. In order to complete these disability evaluations, an IME physician must be qualified by the federal division that administers the program. In these claims, IME physicians usually do not play a role in the determination of diagnostic tests and whether those tests are significant enough to qualify under the rules, but rather are involved when there are issues of causation. Black lung claims can be muddied when there are other comorbid pulmonary diagnoses, such as COPD caused from cigarette smoking or asthma. Since the lifetime benefit awards are usually several hundred thousand dollars, these claims can be contentious.

EEOCIPA is intended to cover those employees of the Department of Energy or its affiliates who develop certain cancers or illnesses from exposure to radiation, beryllium, or silica. The program covers medical expenses and also provides a lump sum compensation award. In these claims, there is usually no role for the IME physician in the area of causation, because the regulations of the act specifically detail what is covered and what is not. There is a role for the IME physician in the area of impairment rating determination as compensation is awarded at a level of $2500 for each 1% impairment. Reapplications are allowed to a claimant if the condition worsens; therefor, the IME physician working with these claims must be very familiar with concepts of apportionment and also needs to be familiar with the internal medicine sections of the *AMA Guides*, which are much less commonly used than the musculoskeletal chapters. Lastly, the EEOCIPA program is unique in that it is the only federal program that uses the fifth edition of the *AMA Impairment Guides* whereas all other programs that require impairment rating determinations mandate use of the sixth edition.

Social Security Disability Programs

The Social Security Administration (SSA) is the largest disability program in the United States and consists of two programs. SSI (Social Security Income) benefits are paid to aged, blind, or disabled claimants with limited financial resources and typically include both a federal and state benefit. Social Security Disability Insurance (SSDI) is a far more commonly known program that is funded through payroll taxes and provides income and medical benefits paid to workers who can no longer work because of a medical disability, to disabled widows of workers, or to a disabled child of a worker who has died, has retired, or is also disabled.

There are two levels where IME physicians can play a substantial role in this system. Most commonly IME physicians may be asked to be a consultative examiner (CE) which is required if the evidence from a claimant's own medical sources

ient to allow a claim examiner to be able to make a qualification deci-
resting twist to SSA CE examinations, however, is that the claimants
ician is actually the preferred source for such an examination. However,
…ed to be conducted by IME physicians because a significant number of treating physicians either do not feel qualified to perform these examinations or prefer not to do them because they have concerns about providing an objective, unbiased opinion.

Individual state agencies who administer the SSDI and SSI programs maintain listings of CE examiners. Thus, if a physician wishes to perform these IMEs, they must contact and register with those offices. Consultative examinations under SSA are focused primarily upon the IME physicians opinion on function and activities of daily living and will require the physician to comment upon the applicants ability to lift, carry, stand, walk, speak, hear, handle objects, etc. There is no other area where medical opinions are necessary as the physician is not expected to comment upon causation or level of impairment. CE examiners do not make the determination on whether the applicant receives the benefits. Instead they are only to communicate the medical information regarding the diagnoses and how they believe those medical problems affect how the applicant is able to perform ADLs. It is at the agency where the determination is made.

It is often stated that SSA consultative examinations are a good way for physicians to start out if they want to add IME services to their practice. CE examinations are typically not contentious, applicants usually present with interesting histories and pathology, and the required reports are comparatively easier and straightforward. Plus, there is usually little chance that the CE will be asked to testify in these cases.

The second level where an IME physician may become involved in the SSDI or SSI process is by becoming a medical expert (ME). MEs provide impartial testimony at ALJ (administrative law judge) hearings and will occasionally be asked to submit answers to questions in writing posed by the judge. Since MEs do not examine claimants, their role is limited to the provision of medical opinions regarding certain medical conditions and their impact upon ADLs. ME testimony is considered along with any other evidence that is presented during a hearing. Similar to the listing of CEs, regional SSA offices maintain a roster of physicians who have agreed to be MEs.

Veterans Administration Entitlement Program

The Department of Veterans Affairs through the Veterans Benefits Administration provides entitlement payments for both service-related disability and medical care to those servicemen and women who received honorable or general discharges and suffered a service-connected disability.

The process that leads to compensation begins when the veteran applies to a regional office. An evaluator at the regional office referred to as a "rater" then reviews the medical claim and submitted information and determines if the veteran is eligible for the benefit. There are clear statutory rules that govern what medical

LTD benefits are usually paid only if the employee is unable to perform the functions of any occupation, and the language regarding the specificity of how this is interpreted is included within each specific policy. Although less common currently, there continue to be individual LTD insurance policies with higher premiums that are considered "own occupation" policies, meaning that benefits are paid when an individual cannot return to their specific prior occupation but may be able to work in other capacities. There are also some LTD policies that pay benefits when an individual has loss of income comparing a prior job that they are no longer able to do to a current job that they are able to do but for which has lower pay.

LTD policies traditionally pay 60% of the individual's prior wage and many have a maximum cap with cost of living allowances. Also, most LTD policies contain a provision that the insured must also concurrently apply for Social Security Disability, and the SSDI entitlements can offset a portion of the wage benefits paid by the LTD carrier.

IME physicians play a role in the LTD decision process usually via the performance of a file review, where an independent evaluator looks at the applicant's medical record and is asked if the medical evidence supports the claim for long-term disability. Usually, each LTD insurance carrier has internal medical professionals who perform initial and confirmatory reviews. Commonly, if the claim is denied, the worker may appeal via the LTD policy language. Often, this appeal will trigger the request for an independent review.

In a few cases, an actual independent examination may be requested. This is typically done when the medical records do not provide a clear picture of the claimant's health status or when there are questions about the legitimacy of certain diagnoses. Commonly, LTD coverage disagreements arise when there are claims of controversial diagnoses or when there are chronic conditions that have episodic exacerbations. Also, mental health claims create the need for IMEs because they are often extremely difficult to analyze based upon treatment records alone.

Lastly, IME physicians may become involved with LTD claims as expert witnesses when a denial of a claim and its appeal has occurred, and the claimant has filed suit against the LTD carrier. Sometimes, these lawsuits involve "bad faith" claims for which the claimant attempts to show that the LTD carrier acted outside of the typical norms during the decision process. These lawsuits are usually quite contentious, are high dollar, and require an IME physician with experience in fitness for duty and knowledge of the bio-psycho-social-economic (BPSE) model of evaluation.

Bibliography

1. National Federation of Independent Business. Workers compensation law—state by state comparison. http://www.nfib.com/content/legal-compliance/legal/workers-compensation-laws-state-by-state-comparison-57181 (2017). Accessed 10 Aug 2017.
2. About OWCP. https://www.dol.gov/owcp/owcpabot.htm (2017). Accessed 10 Aug 2017.
3. Division of Federal Employees Compensation. https://www.dol.gov/owcp/dfec (2017). Accessed 10 Aug 2017.

4. Federal Employees Liability Act. Title 45, U.S. Code Annctated, West Publishing, 51-60.
5. Merchant Marine Act. Title 46 U.S. Code, 688 (1952).
6. Black Lung Benefits Act. https://www.dol.gov/owcp/dcmwc/regs/compliance/blbenact.htm (2017). Accessed 10 Aug 2017.
7. Compensation. https://www.benefits.va.gov/compensation (2017). Accessed 10 Aug 2017.
8. Americas Health Insurance Plans. Guide to disability income insurance. Washington, DC: AHIP; 2009.
9. Benefits for People with Disabilities. https://www.ssa.gov/disability (2017). Accessed 10 Aug 2017.

So You Want to Do IMEs?: How to Develop This Service

3

With the two prior chapters discussing the basics of what an IME is and within what context they are preformed, the remainder of this book will now turn toward a more practical "how to" guide for the physician who wants to add IMEs to their list of services provided or to those physicians who are looking to improve the quality of their IMEs.

I am frequently asked by many colleagues when I lecture or teach at continuing medical education programs "what is the best way for me to get started if I want to do IMEs?"

My traditional response is "it depends"; and as is the case in many situations, the answer lies in the variables of geographic location, type of practice the doctor is currently in, the income goals of the physician, the general legal landscape of the area, and of course supply and demand economics.

Having said that I do have some general guiding principles that I believe can be quite helpful.

Start Simple

If you are brand new to the world of IMEs or perhaps not even sure if this is something you really want to do but want to give it a try, I would strongly suggest beginning with Social Security Comprehensive Examinations (CEs) or Veterans Administration Disability Examinations. The rationale is that these two systems are the least contentious and are relatively straightforward and consistent.

As was previously discussed, VA examinations do not require the IME physician to comment on causation, disability, or impairment. In essence, it requires the IME provider to document the results of the physical examination and to verify the diagnosis. That's it. To me, that is really simple and provides, in my opinion, a reasonable jump off point for beginners. Currently, there is a tremendous shortage of examiners who are willing to do these evaluations. With the increase in the number of claims from veterans from our recent military operations in Afghanistan, Iraq, and elsewhere, the "wounded warrior" applications have skyrocketed.

D.W. Martin, *Independent Medical Evaluation*,
https://doi.org/10.1007/978-3-319-71906-1_3

As of the publication of this book, there are currently four contractors who provide C & P exam services to the VA. They are listed here, with their respective web links. The IME physician should contact these organizations regarding how to register with them and begin to conduct these evaluations. Most, if not all of these contractors, provide educational tools to better prepare the IME physician on the requirements necessary.

- Logistics Health, Inc., La Crosse, Wisconsin
  - www.logisticshealth.com/va
- Medical Support Los Angeles, A Medical Corporation, Pasadena, CA
  - www.mslaca.com/physicians/veterans-provider.php
- QTC Medical Services, Inc., Diamond Bar, California
  - www.qtcm.com
- Veterans Evaluation Services, Inc., Houston, Texas
  - www.vesservices.com

Social Security CEs are also an excellent means for the IME physician to start an IME practice. These evaluations are also straightforward, and the report that is generated follows a standard history and physical examination format familiar to most doctors. In addition, when there is a musculoskeletal complaint, additional range of motion forms are also required to be completed.

What is important for the IME physician to know is that they should, at the conclusion of their report, make specific recommendations regarding the examinee's capabilities and limitations on activities of daily living. Usually, with the paperwork that comes from the respective state jurisdiction that is in charge of scheduling these evaluations, there is a page of instructions that the CE examiner should read in detail, as it provides a bullet point algorithm regarding what information should be addressed within the submitted written report.

In my experience as a CE and as a reader of other CE reports, the quality of the report is a simple reflection of how well the examiner addresses the specifics of the ADL determinations. While it may seem as though it should go without saying, if the CE simply remembers to address each ADL activity that the SSA system demands, they will have no difficulty being able to perform as many of these examinations as they wish. One would be surprised at the number of CE reports that do not drill down to the specific information that is requested.

To begin performing CE examinations, the IME physician should contact their respective state agency that is responsible for maintaining the list of examiners. Sometimes, the state agency will send out information on the SSA disability system, and a few states actually put together reference materials that the examiner may find helpful. For example, the State of Nebraska Disability Determination Services Bureau includes example templates of what a CE report should entail.

One other nicety within the Social Security Disability system is that usually every state agency will provide a dictation service. A toll-free number is given for the CE to use to dictate their reports, and they are then transcribed at the agency's expense and submitted back to the examiner for review and signature. This process reduces the cost burden to the examiner and makes the performance of these exams more financially rewarding.

Having said that, one of the criticisms of the SSA Disability System is that each state may choose the payment level for CEs, and there is quite a bit of variability from state to state. Some states use a "reasonable and customary" fee structure, typically equal to a comprehensive consultative examination or disability evaluation using CPT codes 99245 or 94555, whereas other states may use a discounted Medicare payment schedule for CPT code 99205. As such, there are some states that struggle to find CE examiners because the perception is that the pay is too low, especially when one considers that there is no variability to the fee structure based upon the number of diagnoses or complexity of the medical issues. In other words, CE examiners are paid the same whether one examinee has only a spine condition or whether they have multiple chronic disease states and are taking dozens of medications.

Get Some Training and Education

In Chapter 1, there is a discussion of the various organizations that provide continuing medical education in the area of IME performance. TAKE ADVANTAGE OF THESE OPPORTUNITIES!

I cannot underscore enough how critically important it is to NOT go at this cold turkey! As we said, IME provision is not taught in medical school or residency. Instead, formal medical education focuses only upon treating physician (doctor-patient) relationships. Understanding the role of the IME examiner is thus a fundamentally foreign concept to most physicians, because WE ARE NOT TRAINED TO THINK THIS WAY. My experience in mentoring a number of young IME physicians indicates that it is really difficult for new doctors in practice to be able to end an examination without communicating a treatment plan, prescribing medication, ordering tests, or arranging a follow-up appointment with the examinee. Yet, this is what happens within an IME.

Also, IME physicians tend to struggle with the nuances of the individual different disability systems and their respective requirements. Some of these systems mandate a good understanding of the *AMA Guides to the Evaluation of Permanent Impairment* because calculating impairment rating percentages are required as part of the evaluation. Still other systems require a more focused and scientific attention to issues of causation analysis.

This is where these CME activities become critically important. Each of the listed organizations utilize physician educators with a wealth of experience who are able to articulate, from experience, the information necessary in order to establish competency in these areas. Most of the organizations also provide informal mentorship opportunities whereby a seasoned member of the organization volunteers to be a guide and assist newer physicians by reviewing and critiquing reports and acting as a resource in areas of impairment determination and causation analysis.

I am also often asked how valuable the various certifications and credentials are within these teaching and membership organizations. Again, it depends upon a variety of factors, many of which are not under the control of the IME physician. For a physician who does only a few IMEs or is not interested in expanding their practice with more IMEs, then I do not think these certifications are critical. However if the physician solely performs IMEs or desires to be recognized as an expert in the discipline, then I think it is nearly mandatory; not so much because it is a requirement, but more so as it projects a level of credibility that the IME physician has spent the requisite amount of time on the proper educational areas and have passed an examination that shows a degree of competency. These credentials have a tendency to become more important in litigated cases, where there may be a "dueling doctor phenomenon" where one physician is attempting to be shown as superior to the other in cases where the two physician opinions differ substantially and have important relevance to the case at hand.

Marketing and Advertising

I will admit that I am not big on advertising or marketing IME practices. My feeling on this is that your work in the IME world will have a tendency to market itself.

It needs to be understood that in these disability systems, we have a set of stakeholders that are in reality a small group of people especially when one compares it to other health-care systems. Thus, in my experience, word travels fast, and it is for this reason that I believe word-of-mouth advertising is the best way to increase the number of IME referrals, if that is your goal.

When you start out, if you are performing Social Security CE examinations, the decision-makers at the agency level figure out very quickly who writes a good report and who can be relied upon to communicate to them the information that makes their job easier when determining whether a claimant should be approved or not. What you will find is that a good CE examiner will have no difficulty at all scheduling subsequent evaluations. As a matter of fact, good CE examiners may find themselves turning away exams if their schedules otherwise include other health-care provider activities. This is a nice problem to have.

Once you become a good CE examiner or VA examiner, and if you are in a position to do so, the next level of service usually will come from attorney or insurance carrier requests. How do you get their attention?

It is somewhat easier for the occupational medicine physician to accept requests for IMEs in the workers' compensation system, because that is a system they are already familiar with. In those situations, it may be a simple matter of notifying the various workers' compensation insurance carriers or local employer HR or workers' compensation managers that you are ready to provide these services.

In the work comp insurance world, claims examiners and attorneys often will share a lot of information, and this includes those physicians who provide quality IME work. Here again, we have the word-of-mouth advertising that takes over.

If you are outside the occupational medicine field, you may touch workers compensation cases, for example, if you are an orthopedic surgeon, neurologist, or physiatrist. If this is your situation, the process would be the same as it is for the occ doc; contacting the insurance carrier or local company may be all that is necessary.

What about attorneys? This is a little more difficult in that there are a wide variety of attorney practices, some of which cater more toward plaintiffs and some that cater more toward the defense. Usually, there is a local or county bar association whereby the IME physician can obtain a list of addresses or other contact information of attorneys. A simple letter of introduction about yourself and that you are available for IME referrals will go a long way to opening the door to these types of referrals. Once you have completed a few IMEs, and if they are of good quality, please know that attorneys talk often among themselves both professionally and socially, and once again word-of-mouth advertising will take care of itself.

As has been previously indicated, there are a few disability programs that require an active registration process by the IME physician. Many federal programs require that the physician be placed on a registry or roster of available physicians that can perform the services necessary. This is a relatively easy thing to do, and in many cases you will find that the agency is experiencing a shortage of IME physicians especially for certain types of medical issues. The IME physician might just find that by contacting these agencies, they have created their own niche.

An additional effective marketing strategy is to host an informational event. Some IME physicians invite stakeholders to local or regional lunches or after-hours events that include a short program given by the IME physician regarding what services they can provide. This environment also allows the potential clientele to meet and speak with the IME physician one on one, which is often a fantastic way to promote your testifying skills which are often critical for these relationships to develop.

Yet another mechanism to easily promote your IME practice is to volunteer to write an article for a local newspaper, magazine, or newsletter. You might be surprised to find out how widespread these types of print media are distributed. Chambers of commerce (where business leaders congregate) usually have newsletters or email blurbs that are sent out periodically. Radio and television programs as well as local beat newspaper writers are sometimes looking for "outside the box" stories, and talking with them about what an IME doctor does might be of interest to them. All of these things are essentially levels of free advertising that can pay huge dividends.

Want to improve your testifying skills? A great way to do this is to volunteer to participate in your local or regional law school mock trials and competitions. Not only will this allow you to practice your skills in a nonthreatening environment but also remember that these students might be your next referral sources.

What if you are struggling even after all of the above? You might be in an area where there are many IME providers and the competition might be rough. Or, you might be in an area where you have tried all of the strategies above and you simply are not getting enough referrals to your liking. In these situations, you might consider formal advertising and also contracting with a third-party IME company.

National advertising for IME services is done via several means. One of the teaching organizations I referred to in Chapter 1, SEAK, publishes a national IME directory that is used by many attorneys. There are also other directories that focus on IMEs and expert witnesses that are within the legal profession. Also, obtaining certification or fellowship from the previously described teaching and membership organizations can help as they usually maintain searchable websites where anyone can find a physician with the affiliated credential in a particular area.

Lastly, it is important to address the potential relationships between a physician and third-party (TPA) IME companies. There are a variety of these organizations currently in existence. They were created as a convenient vehicle for insurance carriers, nurse case managers, HR directors, and others to act as a "one stop shop" when an IME is needed. They are of particular help when, for example, an insurance claims representative is dealing with multiple claims in different parts of the country and has neither the time nor the local knowledge to identify a quality local IME provider.

Usually, the TPAs require that the IME physician sign a contract that includes fee agreements, deadlines for report submission, and limits on future involvement such as testimony. I am admittedly equivocal regarding these arrangements. On the one hand, I can see where a struggling IME physician might find these contractual arrangements beneficial if the IME company can guarantee a certain number of examinations so that the IME physician has comfort and confidence that a certain level of business and income stream will come through their doors. One the other hand, I have found some of these companies difficult to work with as they are often uncompromising on points that need reasonable negotiations. Such areas of agreeing to a flat fee regardless of the volume of records to review or the complexity of the case, agreeing on a flat deadline submission (in some cases 48 h after the exam, regardless of the complexity of the case or whether the exam was conducted on a Friday), and acquiescing to a review of your report and deferring to language that the IME company prefers as opposed to your own, can prove challenging.

Also, the business model of these TPAs is to charge their clients a set fee for an IME, reserve a certain percentage of that fee for their business expense and profit, and then pass the residual on to the IME physician. Seasoned IME physicians are left wondering oftentimes why the requesting party has not just contacted their office directly, thereby in some cases saving the requesting party money and increasing the fee realized by the physician. Thus, my suggestion to the IME physician is to consider these opportunities carefully, paying close attention to the details of the contract, and then making a value judgment based upon a cost-benefit analysis of whether or not the relationship is worthwhile.

Bibliography

1. American Board of Independent Medical Examiners. www.abime.org. Accessed 25 Sep 2017.
2. American College of Occupational and Environmental Medicine. www.acoem.org. Accessed 25 Sep 2017.
3. International Academy of Independent Medical Evaluators. www.iaime.org. Accessed 25 Sep 2017.
4. SEAK, Inc. www.seak.com. Accessed 25 Sep 2017.
5. Logistics Health, Inc., La Crosse, WI. www.logisticshealth.com/va. Accessed 7 Jul 2017.

6. Medical Support Los Angeles, A Medical Corporation, Pasadena, CA. www.mslaca.com/physicians/veterans-provider.php. Accessed 07 Jul 2017.
7. QTC Medical Services, Inc., Diamond Bar, CA. www.qtcm.com. Accessed 7 Jul 2017.
8. Veterans Evaluation Services, Inc., Houston, TX. www.vesservices.com. Accessed 7 Jul 2017.
9. Consultative examinations: a guide for health professionals. www.ssa.gov/disability/professionals/greenbook/index.htm (2017). Accessed 7 Jul 2017.

4 Practical Aspects of IME Appointments: Scheduling, Agreements, Etc.

Fantastic. You are now ready to enter the world of IME provision. You have made the decision to add this to the menu of clinical services that you provide. Now what? Does your staff know what an IME is? Does your coding and billing staff know what you are going to charge, how you are going to charge, and what documentation is necessary to charge? Does your scheduler know how much time should be allotted for an IME? There are several areas that you need to pay attention to. It will make your professional life (and the life of your staff) much easier.

The following are areas where clear instructions and understanding need to occur.

How Are IME Appointments Made?

Most IME appointments are initiated by a telephone call from the requesting party. Before you offer this service as part of your practice, you will want to set some basic ground rules. First, you will need to decide how many IMEs you want to do. Some physicians have only IME practices. Others include IMEs as part of a larger menu of services.

Most physicians who are novices to IMEs usually will want to start slow until they have a better handle on the process and get comfortable with the dynamics of the evaluation protocols. We suggest that you start by scheduling no more than one IME per day. Once you become more efficient, you can then increase the number of evaluations per day scheduled to what you feel comfortable with.

Physicians will also want to review the required information that will need to be gathered by the individual who is responsible for fielding telephone calls and setting up appointments. Since the dynamics of the IME process are a bit unique, usually this is a task that is reserved for only seasoned receptionists or an office manager, someone who is knowledgeable about your expectations and the differences that an IME appointment will require compared to others.

During the initial telephone conversation, information should be gathered concerning the name, address, and contact information of the requesting party as well

D.W. Martin, *Independent Medical Evaluation*,
https://doi.org/10.1007/978-3-319-71906-1_4

as the name, address, and contact information of the person who is going to be examined. It is also important to identify the system under which the IME is being requested; in other words, is the evaluation to be conducted under the guise of the workers' compensation system, a personal injury lawsuit, or some other system?

Once that basic information is gathered, the individual responsible for making the appointment should then ask about the amount of medical or other records that will be sent that will need to be reviewed. A word of caution about this step is that many requesting parties surprisingly do not know the amount. However, in my experience, it is best to press the requestor for at least some ballpark number, as it is difficult to make an appointment based upon an assumption that there are only a few records to review and then find that the FedEx delivery man has used a two-wheel cart to bring in the two boxes of records to review later in the week! Obviously, garnering information on the number of records needed to be reviewed will allow the scheduler to set aside the proper amount of time needed for the physician to review them prior to the examination.

It is also important at this initial contact stage that any information regarding your individual requirements or expectations be communicated up front with the requesting party. Such issues would include expectations on how soon the examinee is expected to appear at the examiner's office (some examiners require the examinee to appear several minutes ahead of the actual appointment time to complete necessary paperwork, complete history forms, etc., while other examiners "build in" to their appointment times this process. For example, an appointment might be set for 1:00 p.m. with the office staff full well knowing that the first 30 min is set aside for preliminary form completion and other tasks and that the physician will only start their encounter at 1:30 p.m.). Other items to discuss at this point so that there are no misunderstandings would be things such as no-show policies, expectations for when the report is to be completed, any possible prepayment or deposit requirements, and if there is any expectation for the requesting party to speak with the evaluating physician either before or after the examination or both.

Once all this information is gathered, a preliminary appointment time can be set and given to the requesting party, and it is explained that a written and signed acknowledgement letter will need to be sent out and returned prior to the appointment being confirmed.

How Are IME Appointments Confirmed?

Once the initial telephone contact has occurred and a tentative appointment has been made, the physician should send out a confirmation letter to the requesting party that will need to be initialed or signed and returned to the physician's office for the appointment to be confirmed. This is a recommended methodology that cannot be underscored enough as this process will eliminate much disagreement, confusion, and misunderstandings when verbal communication can break down.

Within this confirmation letter, the IME physician includes the date and time of the appointment and the name of the examinee with the examinee's contact information. Also, in this confirmation letter, the "rules" or expectations of the physician are communicated with respect to no-shows, cancellations, the sending of records, expectations for report completion, and finally billing. Although not necessarily considered a binding contract, this confirmation letter sets the ground rules for the evaluation process and sets protection parameters for the IME physician.

Additionally, the IME physician's office should send out a different confirmation letter to the examinee. This letter is intended to verify the appointment time, location, and duration. This letter does not have to be long and is often a complementary letter in that the requesting party also will typically have communication with the examinee regarding the appointment dynamics. Many IME physicians elect to communicate to the examinee in this letter a general explanation of the type of examination and also any expectations. It is generally a good practice to explain that the IME appointment may last longer than a typical physician appointment and that the examinee should refrain from bringing family members, especially children, with them to the appointment. Nothing is more difficult than having the examinee trying to corral three small children in an exam room while an IME is being done, and some IME physicians have rules about this that are mainly borne out of liability concerns. When asked about this type of a policy, I simply explain that I am not in the day care business and that my clinic has no ability to provide for child care during the IME appointment time. Also, I explain that to do a thorough and complete history and physical examination, it is important that both the examinee and examiner are not distracted.

In the following section, we will review common areas that you will want to make sure that you include in your confirmation letter and for which you will want to establish as your IME policy.

There are examples of a confirmation letter for both the requesting party and the examinee that are at the end of this chapter. Additionally, I have included a copy of the current "rule sheet" that I send out with the confirmation letter to the requesting party. Please note that I have also included information on impairment rating examinations, MMI examinations, and second opinion evaluations. While these are not IMEs because of the fact that a doctor-patient relationship is established with these services, the rules are included for completeness and for your benefit of being able to compare and contrast them.

Issues to Consider When Determining Reasonable IME Provision Policy

Expectation for Record Receipt

Determining when the records need to be in the physician's office for review is probably less important in the electronic age than it was several years ago. However, there will need to be time scheduled out prior to the IME to review records. Most physicians prefer to review records shortly before the IME, some the same day. We suggest no greater than 1 or 2 days in advance. As a result, the records should be in the possession of the physician's office preferably at least by the day prior to when they are to be reviewed. Some IME physicians indicate within their policies that a no-show fee will be charged if this deadline is not met, which is probably a good practice. Obviously, if the records are not in the possession of the IME physician when time is scheduled out to review them, it necessitates re-scheduling the IME to a later date.

Cancellation Policy

The IME physician is wise to consider what a reasonable cancellation policy will be. With the IME appointment typically being at least an hour in length, most physicians are unable to recover the lost time and lost billing revenue if these appointments are cancelled soon before the appointment date. Another consideration is how will the situation be handled when time was set aside to review the records (especially if they are voluminous) only to then have the appointment cancelled. Although practices certainly vary depending upon the type of practice that the physician has, we suggest that a cancellation that occurs less than 5 working office days prior to the appointment be assessed either a cancellation or no-show fee. As a general guide, this cancellation fee should be set at a level of a minimum of 50% or one half of the minimum IME fee up to the maximum of what the original charge would have been if there were no cancellation. We have found the 50% fee level to be reasonable for a physician who has a healthy practice that provides other services.

No-Show Policy

Just as is the case with a cancellation, the IME physician should be firm with a reasonable no-show policy. Again, the physician simply cannot recover the lost time and lost revenue when the IME examinee simply does not show for the appointment. Like the cancellation fee, we suggest a minimum of 50% of what the minimum IME fee would be, however, it is also important to consider here the situation when time has been spent in reviewing records prior to the appointment. Some physicians in this situation also bill the lost record review time in addition to the no-show fee, which is reasonable to do especially if the amount of records required multiple hours to review and even more so if there is little expectation that the appointment will be rescheduled.

Within the no-show policy should also be a statement concerning what is considered what are called "late arrivals" or "late shows." This is the situation when the examinee arrives for their appointment but is late doing so. Each IME physician will need to determine what is reasonable and what is not, but I have instituted a 20-min rule; in my policy, an examinee is considered a "no-show" also if they are greater than 20 min late for their appointment and are not seen. Of course, this is information that is included in both the confirmation letters to the requesting party and also to the examinee.

Interpreter Services

IME physicians will often be faced with evaluating a non-English speaking examinee. It is absolutely critical in these situations to have confidence that an interpreter is doing a good job. Thus, it is recommended that a certified interpreter be used, because many times IMEs are then subject to legal proceedings. There are interpretation agencies that are in existence in order to accomplish exactly what is needed; to provide an impartial interpreter who can be relied upon to communicate accurate and consistent information back and forth between physicians and examinee.

In all cases, the fee and scheduling of the interpreter should be the responsibility of the requesting party. It is recommended to avoid telephonic services such as what is available through communication companies and internet service providers. Not only can telephonic services lack the professionalism and consistency necessary for these examinations, but often times the individual providing the service over the telephone is not available in the future if a legal question arises and often they are not agreeable to partaking in medicolegal evaluations in the first place.

It is therefore critical that in the confirmation letter sent to the requesting party, and also as part of the standard IME policy of the physician, that there is some information regarding details surrounding the use of interpreters. Also, it should include the fact that if an interpreter no-shows or is late for the appointment, that this is the responsibility of the requesting party and not the IME physician, and as such, late or no-show interpreters can also cause a no-show fee to occur.

Report Deadlines

Expectations regarding how quickly an IME report can be generated after the examination vary greatly across the country and span the spectrum of the various different disability systems. Some systems, such as state workers compensation systems, may have a report deadline of only a few days. This is also the practice of many of the so-called IME "brokers"; companies that contract out for IME services and act as a third party or "go between" the requesting party and physician. In these situations, if there is statute or contractual agreement that sets this, then it should also be stated in this manner within the IME physician policy and their confirmation letter. However, many IMEs are under no such legal deadline. In these situations, we have found that a ten-working-day report deadline is looked upon favorably by most requesting parties and is also reasonable for most physicians. On a side note, many hospital systems (such as mine) have physician policies that address timeliness expectations or medical staff policy rules regarding record completion. If you are a physician that is bound to those rules, then IME reports would more than likely fall under these rules. It just so happens that my hospital system has a ten-working-day record completion policy, which fits nicely with my predetermined self-imposed reasonable report deadline.

Prepayment Requirements or "Deposits"

Some IME physicians require that a requesting party provide a prepayment deposit to schedule an IME appointment. The practice typically is used when the physician has either had experiences where bills have not been paid for IME services of which there have been disagreements about the amount that has been billed.

When this practice is used, the usual course of events is that the requesting party asks for an appointment. The appointment is then "held" or preliminarily placed on the IME physician's schedule, but only confirmed once the deposit or prepayment has been received (and in most cases when it has cleared the bank). If this procedure is adopted, it is important for the IME physician to include within their policy a rule as to how long an appointment may be held before it is released. Obviously, the appointment time should not be left taken if the deposit has not appeared. A usual time frame is to require the deposit to be in hand within 10 days of the appointment which allows another few days to make sure that the payment clears the bank. Some policies require cashier's checks or electronic guarantee payments, which, of course, avoids the necessity of waiting on a bank to ensure that the funds are indeed available.

In my 20-plus-year career of IME provision, I have never instituted a prepayment or deposit rule. Whether it is because of a more conservative Midwestern perspective or the fact that I work for a large hospital system, I have never been "stiffed" on an IME bill; thus the process of requiring a deposit has never been necessary. However, I am aware of colleagues in other locations who have indeed had to resort to means such as the use of collection agencies and even going to small claims court in order to have their bill paid. Most have indicated to me that their bills have not been paid because either the report or opinion that was generated was not thought to be helpful for the client or examinee or that the requesting party was not reputable (usually small fly-by-night lawyers who were grasping at straws trying to obtain a medical opinion that was contradictory to science or best practices).

Billing

What is a reasonable rate for an IME? This is a question that is asked not only of me but of other stakeholders quite frequently. My answer is that it is typically a function of supply and demand economics of the geographic location where the physician practices.

In some cases, IMEs that are performed under certain benefit systems or jurisdictions are subject to fee schedules. This is common, for example, for Social Security Disability evaluations where the state agency in charge of obtaining a Comprehensive Examination (CE) may have a statutory fee that can only be paid at a certain rate for the service. Some state workers compensation systems also might limit the IME fees.

However, in most personal injury cases and in most workers compensation systems, there are no statutory limits. IME physicians typically determine their charges based upon what a standard and fair rate is within their practice location. Fees can also vary depending upon specialty, and there is a trend toward higher fees when IMEs are performed by surgical subspecialists.

The methodology of IME billing is best accomplished using a time-based fee approach. I suggest that the IME physician establish a baseline or minimum charge that encompasses 2 hours of time, usually divided into 1 hour of record review and report generation and 1 hour devoted to taking the history and performing the physical examination. Additional charges can then be made if the case takes longer than the standard baseline 2 hours of time. Although practices vary, a common method is to bill for each additional 30-minute increment above and beyond the standard baseline rate.

Proper analysis of the market for IMEs and establishment of fee rates are specific to the practice, geographical location, specialty of the physician, and in some cases the level of expertise and experience. The IME physician will want to make sure that they charge at a level at least to the degree that other evaluation and management services within the scope of their practices dictate for approximately the same amount of professional time spent, but in most cases, significantly higher than what the level 5 E&M service billing is as IMEs are specialized services that go beyond the typical scope and expertise that this level of service establishes. Some colleagues have indicated that they feel that the baseline IME charge should be on the order of triple what the typical level 5 payment is for a new encounter.

Experiences with proper fee identification indicate that the IME physician can usually determine whether their fees are too high or too low based upon the requests that are taken. If the phone rings off the hook and it is difficult to accommodate all the appointment requests, chances are that the IME physician should raise their rates. If, however, there are few phone calls, then chances are the rates are too high and need to be adjusted. There are some organizations that provide survey data on IME charges that can be easily found using an internet search engine. Caution should be given when using these data sets as often there is not enough statistically significant survey returns given for a certain geographical area or practice specialty.

Along with setting a fee schedule for IMEs, the physician should also think about a fee schedule for other ancillary professional services that naturally derive from this. Medical testimony, attorney consultation, and scientific or medical research time are items that also need to have appropriate fees set for their respective activities.

If you happen to work in a clinic or other setting that is required to use CPT codes and you happen to be paid based upon RVUs, then that is often times a difficult situation if you want to add IMEs to your repertoire. Although the American Medical Association CPT coding system does list appropriate CPT codes for IME and its associated medicolegal services, CMS (Center for Medicare and Medicaid Services) does not assign an RVU (relative value unit) to these codes. As a result, physicians who are paid based upon a dollar multiplier per the number of RVUs generated over a certain period of time will want to make sure that an agreed upon, often negotiated, yet "made up" RVU value is assigned to these services. In this case, make sure that you are negotiating from a perspective that little physician office overhead is actually used for IME services. Remember, there is no special equipment needed; there is no treatment, and there is little to no nursing activity. Essentially, the overhead consists of staff time required to make the appointments and send out and receive the confirmation letters, costs of having an exam room, and whatever transcription or hardware/software expenses are involved in generating the report.

An example CPT billing menu of services is included at the end of this chapter. Some of the CPT codes are modified or "dummy codes" that are specific to my situation that I have created due to need for specificity concerning some of the physician activities that I perform. There are other models, but these are provided as but one example for consideration.

How Long Should IME Appointments Be?

As we have suggested a methodology of reviewing the medical records prior to the examination, the issue of proper time scheduling becomes critical. When one determines the amount of medical records to review, the proper time can be committed to that task. At a minimum, 1 hour should be set aside to review medical records in advance of the appointment time. I am frequently asked the question "how many pages can I expect to review in an hour?" This is a tricky question to answer, because the content and quality of information in the records varies greatly. For example, if you are going to review a deposition transcript, these pages are dense with verbiage and will take quite a bit longer to review. On the other hand, you may have a considerable number of pages from a hospitalization where an electronic record system is used and you very well may find that your eyes glaze over 65 pages into the nursing care documentation which probably has no relevance to what you are evaluating. Regardless, you are probably going to make some errors in estimating this when you first start doing IMEs, but that is okay….you will eventually develop a pattern that will work well for you. But, at least to give you some guidance, I have found that it is reasonable to canvass 300–350 pages of records in an hour. If you do the math, that is about five pages per minute. While you might think that is going pretty quick, you will also find that once you start this process that there will be some record duplication and redundancy.

Regarding scheduling the evaluation, in general, a minimum of 1 hour will be needed to conduct a thorough history and physical examination. Depending upon the complexity of the medical problems that need to be evaluated as well as the need to address multiple organ systems, this may require a longer period. The suggestion is to obtain as much information up front regarding these complexities and adjust the length of the scheduled appointment time if necessary.

As you can see from the discussion above, a minimum 2-hour time frame is the suggested scheduling recommendation for an IME that will include the record review and the examination.

How Much Time Do You Need to Craft the IME Report?

Once you have completed the examination and reviewed the records, it is now time to create your report. Most IME physicians elect to create the report soon after the examination is completed; some directly afterward, some later the same day and sometimes if the report will be lengthy a few days later. While I have heard of some physicians waiting even weeks later to create the report, it must be understood that it is a best practice to craft the report as soon after the examination as possible.

There are several advantages to this practice. Obviously, the requesting parties will be happier with you if you do this on the same day because the final report can be sent out only a day or two after the exam is completed. However, the most significant advantage is that the IME physician will have a better recollection of all the relevant examination information if the report is generated right after the examination. Let us be honest, everyone, including physicians, loses memory or recall of information as time passes. Even though you might be a meticulous notetaker, you are not going to be able to record everything.

How Are IME Reports and Records Handled?

Most IME physicians either use a transcriptionist service or some sort of voice recognition software to create their reports. The attention to detail and the fact that the IME report is subject to medicolegal scrutiny means that electronic health record systems (also called "EHRs," electronic medical records (EMRs), or, for those who believe they have not really improved patient care, electronic billing records (EBRs)) that use templates and point-and-click methodologies are not conducive to creating these.

If a voice recognition software package is used for report generation, and the IME physician is not familiar with them but wishes to go that route, they should plan for a considerable amount of time in setting up their system. All of these software programs incorporate a "learning phase" within which the software "learns" your voice pitch, phrase speed, etc. But, you should also plan on spending a significant amount of time in creating proper titles, subheadings, and formatting structures that are typically unique to IME reports. We will address the report and its intricacies in more detail and also provide examples of reports in Chapter 9.

Once the report is generated and sent out, the IME physician is recommended to keep a copy of the report and any records and correspondence regarding the IME. Although a formal IME recordkeeping standard does not exist, there may be certain jurisdictional rules that will dictate how long the report and records need to be kept. In some jurisdictions, it might be acceptable to return the records to the requesting party with the report wherein no recordkeeping responsibilities exist for the IME physician. When in doubt, it is best to keep both the report and the records in perpetuity. I can cite many examples where this practice has proven beneficial. One example is when an IME examinee has a later claim and a different representative is trying to find any prior records. You may find yourself the only source of medical records if the subsequent claim has happened several years later. While it might seem tedious to store records forever, I have found that it actually pays dividends because you often are the "last hope" of many parties who are trying to find them.

My strong suggestion is to store your reports and records electronically. Trying to save paper is tedious, costly, and sometimes backbreaking (literally) if you store them in boxes in a storage facility. When doing so, scanning is the best method. Investing in a high-speed scanner is not really a suggestion but a requirement. Be advised that it is always prudent to have a backup method for your electronic storage, either in a dedicated hard drive separate from your first storage area or using some cloud-based option.

What Happens If There Are Additional Requests or Inquiries That Are Received After the IME Is Completed?

You may encounter a situation where the requesting party asks an additional question or needs more clarification regarding an opinion that you have given within your report. The IME physician should be prepared for this situation and have a plan on how to address it. Additional inquiries should not be looked upon as difficulties or in a negative way. Rather, requesting parties may not be aware of certain realities of a given injury or illness claim or may need to drill down on some finer points of items such as the history or the physical examination.

When these requests occur, time should be set aside in the IME physician's schedule to review the additional questions. Sometimes, additional record information is sent that often reflects more recent health-care encounters which typically the IME physician will discover during their interview of the examinee. Appropriate time should be set aside to review these additional records.

Often, all the requesting party may want to know is "does the review of the additional medical records change your opinion in your IME report?" This is a simple and relatively straightforward task. But in other situations, multiple and more complex questions may be asked.

When providing added reviews or opinions, it is important for the IME physician to state that the follow-up response needs to be considered an addendum to the original IME. Doing so makes it specifically clear to any reader that the follow-up letter or report is not intended to stand on its own; instead it is an extension of the original IME report. Also, it should be noted that the same parameters regarding the follow-up or addendum remain in force.

Appendix 1: Example Confirmation Letter for Requesting Party

September 24, 2017

XYZ Insurance Company
Mr. George Zazzy
420 Roller Street
Hightown, CO 88878

RE: Independent Medical Examination of Constance C Chronicus

Dear Mr. Zazzy:

Thank you for your telephone call from this morning wherein we have tentatively scheduled the above individual for an Independent Medical Examination that will be conducted by Douglas W Martin MD on Friday October 9, 2017 at 3:00 p.m.

With your signature below, you have acknowledged the fee schedule and parameters surrounding the IME set forth in the accompanying documents.

If you have any questions, please contact us.

Sincerely,

Kara Benny
Office Manager

Acknowledged and agreed:

______________________________ ____________________

Mr. Goerge Zazzy Date

Please fax back to 712-444-4000

Appendix 2: Example Confirmation Letter to Examinee

September 24, 2017

Ms. Constance C Chronicus
8675309 Jenny Avenue
Tutone, CO 87958

RE: Your Upcoming Independent Medical Examination of October 9, 2017

Dear Ms. Chronicus:

You have been scheduled for an independent medical examination (IME) to be conducted by Douglas W Martin MD on Friday October 9, 2017 at our office.

We ask that you arrive at 2:30 p.m.

Please note that this examination will last approximately 90 minutes.

Please contact us at least 48 hours in advance if you will be unable to make your appointment and an attempt will be made to reschedule. Arriving late for your appointment unfortunately cannot be accommodated.

We ask that you plan ahead regarding travel and that you bring only one friend or family member with you if you so choose. Our office is unable to accommodate child care or supervision.

If you have any questions, please contact us as soon as possible. We look forward to seeing you on October 9.

Sincerely,

Kara Benny
Office Manager

Appendix 3: Example List of IME and Other Rules to Be Sent with Requesting Party Letter

Protocols and Policies: Medicolegal Clinic Services

Independent Medical Examinations

1. All examinations shall be scheduled for one hour, unless the complexity of the case demands a longer appointment time.
2. All pertinent medical records shall arrive at least 48 hours prior to the scheduled appointment.

3. All pertinent x-rays shall arrive at least 48 hours prior to the scheduled appointment.
4. The collection, assimilation, and distribution of the medical records and x-rays are the responsibility of the party requesting the exam.
5. A cover letter detailing any special requests or questions to be answered is recommended.
6. The basic clinical charge for the exam, record review, and report generation is not set by Dr. XXX but is set by administration. The basic charge includes one hour for the examination and one hour for record review and report generation. Any additional time needed will be charged at an additional rate, set by administration for each additional 30 minute increment.
7. Any cancellation less than 48 hours prior to the appointment will necessitate a "no-show" fee set by administration.
8. If an examinee does not show for the appointment or is greater than 20 (twenty) minutes late for the examination, this will incur the no-show fee. Please understand that it is typical for most IME examinations to take one hour and that being late can significantly impact the day-to-day operations of the clinic.

Impairment Rating Examinations/Finalization Examinations

1. All examinations shall be scheduled for one hour, unless the complexity of the case demands a longer appointment time.
2. These examinations are defined as impairment evaluations and finalization appointments on patients that Dr. XXX has cared for that need impairment ratings and/or permanent return to work prescriptions (restrictions) that go above and beyond the normal follow-up examination.
3. A cover letter is recommended from the requesting party to insure that all issues are addressed by Dr. XXX.
4. Due to the increasing frequency of no-shows for these appointments, a no-show policy will be implemented.
5. The typical charge for this examination is not set by Dr. XXX but is set by administration and is a flat fee, unless there are circumstances where additional time is needed for the examination or record procurement above the normal one-hour time allotment.
6. Any cancellation less than 48 hours prior to the appointment will necessitate a "no-show" fee also set by administration.
7. If an examinee does not show for the appointment or is greater than 20 (twenty) minutes late for the examination, this will incur the no-show fee. Please understand that it is typical for most of these examinations to take one hour and that being late can significantly impact the day-to-day operations of the clinic.

Second Opinion Examinations

1. Please understand that there are two basic types of second opinion examinations, those where opinion alone is desired and those where there is an assumption of treatment. It is absolutely imperative that the type of exam be explicitly communicated to the clinic in advance of the appointment.
2. Second opinion examinations are intended for those injured employees who have already sought treatment from other providers for their workers compensation

claim. Typically, second opinion examinations cover treatment recommendations alone, and do not rise to the level of determining impairment or disability as in an independent medical examination.

3. All examinations shall be scheduled for one hour, unless the complexity of the case demands a longer appointment time.
4. All pertinent medical records shall arrive at least 48 hours prior to the scheduled appointment.
5. All pertinent x-rays shall arrive at least 48 hours prior to the scheduled appointment.
6. The collection, assimilation, and distribution of the medical records and x-rays are the responsibility of the party requesting the exam.
7. A cover letter detailing any special requests or questions to be answered is recommended.
8. The charge for these examinations will follow the CPT codes and applicable fees for the complexity of the case.
9. Due to the increasing frequency of no-shows for these appointments, a no-show policy will be implemented.
10. Any cancellation less than 48 hours prior to the appointment will necessitate a "no-show" fee that is not set by Dr. Martin, but is set by administration.
11. If an examinee does not show for the appointment or is greater than 20 (twenty) minutes late for the examination, this will incur the no-show fee. Please understand that it is typical for most of these examinations to take one hour and that being late can significantly impact the day-to-day operations of the clinic.

Depositions

1. All depositions shall be scheduled at least two weeks prior. A minimum of two hours will be scheduled for all depositions.
2. All deposition will occur at Dr. XXX's office @ Anyplace, USA unless other arrangements are made. A conference room that includes a speaker phone is available to accommodate.
3. All depositions cancelled less than 5 working days prior to their occurrence will be subject to charge at the regular deposition fee rate. The rate is not set by Dr. XXX, but is set by administration.
4. Charges for depositions shall originate from the originally scheduled time for the beginning of the deposition. Late appearances of attorneys or recorders are not the responsibility of the physician.

Testimony

1. In-person testimony is available for workers compensation, personal injury, and professional liability cases.
2. Scheduling of such testimony shall occur at least two weeks in advance, sooner if possible.
3. Usually, testimony is scheduled for one-half day blocks, but may be scheduled for a shorter period or longer period of time depending upon the complexity of the case.

4. The charge for live testimony is not set by Dr. XXX but is set by administration. There is a base rate for the first hour and then an additional rate at 30 minute increments following.
5. The hourly amount will be calculated from the time of departure from the clinic to include travel time to the destination of testimony and include return travel time. The billed time will include only the time that is part of normally scheduled clinic time.
6. Any travel expenses above and beyond driving expenses will be the responsibility of the requesting party.
7. All testimony cancelled less than 5 working days prior to its occurrence will be subject to charge at the regular deposition fee rate.

Appendix 4: Example CPT Codes Used

IME

99456—Work related or medical disability examination by other than the treating physician that includes:

- Completion of a medical history commensurate with the patient's condition
- Performance of an examination commensurate with the patient's condition
- Formulation of a diagnosis, assessment of capabilities and stability, and calculation of impairment
- Development of future medical treatment plan
- Completion of necessary documentation/certificates and report

Impairment or Disability Evaluation—Current Patient

99455—Same as above—difference is only that this applies to a current patient where a doctor-patient relationship has already been established

99499—Unlisted Evaluation and Management Service

Some systems use 99499 for a variety of items that cannot be categorized elsewhere

99075—Medical Testimony

Independent File Reviews

99080—Special reports such as insurance forms, more than the information conveyed in the usual medical communications or standard reporting form

Some systems use 99080 for a variety of items that are not well categorized by other CPT codes such as narrative responses to letters from insurance carriers, HR managers, etc. and other correspondence generated by the physician

Bibliography

1. Brigham C. Common tips for IMEs (Part 1) Perfecting the IME process. Guides Newsletter. 2000 Sep/Oct.
2. Brigham C, Ensalada L. Common tips for IMEs (Part 1) Perfecting the IME process: pre-evaluation. Guides Newsletter. 2000 Sep/Oct.
3. Blair B. IME bootcamp. Proceedings of the 27th Annual Meeting and Scientific Session of the American Academy of Disability Evaluating Physicians; 2014 Jan 9; San Antonio. Chicago: AADEP.

5 Setting the Stage: What You Can Learn (and Not) from the Medical Records and How to Use Them

Cover Letters

Once the IME appointment has been made and all parties have been notified regarding the expectations and parameters within which the examination will be conducted, the referring source will send a cover letter. Referral sources who are more experienced in dealing with these cases will usually provide a summary of the claim, a brief explanation of the medical problems, and questions that they need answered by the IME physician.

In some cases, the IME physician will not receive a cover letter. This is a poor practice, in so much as the IME physician is then left to ponder what the medical issues are that the referring source is questioning and has no reference point regarding the background of the claim. It is recommended that the IME physician require a cover letter form the referral source so as to avoid any misperceptions. Well-crafted cover letters will include a listing of specific questions typically placed at the end of the letter. This should be the focal point of the IME physician at the beginning of the evaluative process, which really begins here and is followed by a review of the past records sent by the referral source.

Protocols for Reviewing Records

Earlier in my career, I encountered fellow IME physicians who stated to me that they preferred to not look at previous medical records until AFTER they had completed their independent medical examination. I could never quite understand that perspective. They indicated to me that they did it this way because they felt that they would be biased in some way if they read the records before they completed their own history and physical examination.

While I can understand that concern on a certain level, I don't agree with that practice. Rather, I think it is critical to obtain and review as many past medical records in advance of the IME examination. A review of the records can provide a

D.W. Martin, *Independent Medical Evaluation*,
https://doi.org/10.1007/978-3-319-71906-1_5

solid background for the contextual questions that require the focus of the IME physician. I cannot imagine conducting an IME evaluation without having previously looked at the records. To me, this would necessitate more generalized historical questions to be asked which would take more time; time that is precious to the evaluator and also time that is important to the examinee.

A prior analysis of the treatment records gives the IME physician a chronological viewpoint of the treatment of the medical condition from the start to the present. It allows the IME physician the ability to drill down on more questionable or debatable portions of the record. It narrows the IME physician's history to those questions posed to the examinee that will clearly show where the issues lie. Many times it is interesting to find that the information that the examinee THOUGHT they heard from their treating providers is not consistent with what is communicated in the medical record. It is often times the job of the IME physician to determine WHY this is. When there is disparity in the record compared to the history given by the examinee, is this a simple mistake? Is it because the examinee is fabricating the information? Is the treating physician purposefully not disclosing information in the written record that was verbalized to their patient? These are all questions for which the IME physician is to attempt to resolve, at least to the best of their ability. One could not possibly do this without previously reviewing the medical records relevant to the case at hand.

It is suggested that the IME physician have a standard mechanism or protocol for reviewing records. This is most helpful in cases where there are hundreds if not thousands of pages to evaluate. It is a recommendation that the IME doctor have an agreement or at least a conversation with the requesting source as to how best to send the prior records. In cases where there are significant numbers, electronic transmission may be more practical. However, some IME physicians prefer paper records no matter what the circumstance, so that they can file, group, categorize, and compare in ways that work for them.

Regardless of the means of transmission, the IME physician should know that the requesting party may transmit records by indexing or "tabbing" in different ways. A common practice is to place all treatment records form the same source (e.g., from the same doctor, same therapist, same hospital) together, each source having its own tab or index. Other practices might use a strict chronological order, where the records are put in order by date of service. It seems that the former practice is easier and more practical and provides ease of understanding as to how the individual treating source is thinking through the problem along the continuum of time. Problems with the chronological method include the fact that the medical issues may be difficult to follow, especially in cases where multiple providers are involved at the same time. Also, there are differences in chronological sorting in that some referral sources will put records together with the oldest record on top, whereas other sources will put the most recent records at the front. Regardless of methodology, the IME physician should communicate their preference in advance; most referral sources are willingly able to accommodate such requests.

Once the records are organized in a manner preferable to the IME physician, a careful and detailed review should occur. It is helpful in this process to take notes that can be referred to either at the time of the examination and/or when the report is generated. Taking notes and writing down questions proves to be useful as it also helps the IME physician to focus on the issues that the referral source is questioning.

Specific attention should be paid to points in time when major diagnostics or interventions are performed. Noting the dates of MRI scans and surgical procedures are very important. In cases where fitness for duty or return to work is debatable, the IME physician should note when treating physicians have changed their recommendations on work status and the rationale (if it is discussed) for the placement of temporary or permanent restrictions.

I always look for inconsistencies in the record. Most often, one can predict where the contentious issues of a claim reside by identifying in the record where these exist. When these are found, it should serve as a reminder to the IME physician to expand the history taking on those subjects when the examination occurs.

In musculoskeletal claims, I frequently pay very close attention to physical and occupational therapy notes. It is my belief that often these records are not paid attention to at the level they deserve. Commonly, you will see the PT or OT comment upon activity or work issues at these appointments that are either cursorily or not addressed at the physician appointments. One also can obtain a clearer picture of function from OT and PT documentation than in other medical encounter documentation. Lastly, OT and PT evaluations are very good and identifying trends over a series of visits and can paint a picture regarding delayed recovery or maximum recovery.

To help the IME physician further, it is helpful to keep in mind that eventually the evaluator will be telling a story when it comes time for the IME report to be written. Storytelling is often an art form, but when combing through the records, ask yourself if can tell a good story by what is contained within them. If you can, great, then you have probably done a good job. If not, you may have missed something, and this should trigger a rereview in an attempt to fill in the missing information. Sometimes, though, you will not be able to tell a good story. This is when you will need to try to complete the puzzle by asking the right questions of the claimant during the history-taking portion of the examination.

Nonmedical Records Including Surveillance

Referral sources will sometimes include nonmedical records for the IME physician to review. When there has been an accident, photographs or maps of the areas where the injuries occurred can be very helpful. Witness statements sometimes can disclose information that the examinee does not or may help to provide better clarity on the events that occurred. With the increased popularity of security cameras, it is common now for the IME physician to be sent a video file of a recording of the accident itself.

Other nonmedical records may be sent that are given in an attempt to help fill in ancillary information that the referral source believes helpful in the evaluation process. Employment records that include attendance, discipline, or leave requests are sometimes included and are argued by the referral source as evidence of potentially poor work performance which may translate into illness behavior. Historical records of legal involvement including arrest records and listings of prior medicolegal claims are forwarded when there are concerns of inappropriate claim behavior or overt malingering.

With the advent of and increasing use of social media, claimant postings to Facebook, Twitter, Instagram, and others are now sometimes also included within records to be reviewed. These can be helpful to understand claims of disability and are often sent by referral sources to show that medically imposed activity restrictions are either not followed or are incorrectly assigned.

Surveillance videos, often times recorded by private investigation firms, are forwarded to the IME physician by referral sources in an attempt to show that the claimant typically has a higher level of functional capabilities than what they are claiming or by what has been imposed by their treating physician. Private investigation firms can be quite ingenious with hidden cameras and methods that they use to obtain these types of footage. I have witnessed cameras inside baseball caps, attached to grocery store carts, contained within sunglasses, and even within a patch on a Scouting uniform.

Caution should be used when reviewing these nonmedical records. It is recommended that when the IME physician renders opinions on medical issues that these opinions should be based upon medical information. While it is true that these nonmedical sources can provide background information and give the evaluator a "flavor" for the validity of the medical claim, medical opinions cannot and should not ever be based solely on these nonmedical items. One last comment: make sure to the best of your ability that the person on a surveillance video is actually the person that you are examining. I have personally been involved in evaluating a claim where the private investigator filmed the wrong person, the claimant's twin brother.

Bibliography

1. Brigham C. Referral letter for the performance of an independent medical evaluation. Guides Newsletter. 2005 Jan/Feb.
2. Blair B. IME bootcamp. Proceedings of the 27th Annual Meeting and Scientific Session of the American Academy of Disability Evaluating Physicians; 2014 Jan 9; San Antonio. Chicago: AADEP.

Taking an IME History and Conducting the Examination

6

Prior to the history, the IME physician will have reviewed pertinent past medical and other records that would have been forwarded by the referral source. After reading the referral letter, the evaluator should have a reasonably good idea as to the areas of the history that need to be explored further.

I advocate for approaching every IME with a certain set of core principles which I refer to as the "4 Cs" that stand for:

Clarification of purpose
Complete preparation
Content
Communication

Of these, the first three will be discussed in detail in this chapter. A significant portion of communication will be covered in Chapter 9 that speaks to the development and writing of the IME report.

Clarification of Purpose

Clarification of purpose refers to the preparatory measures that need to occur prior to the examination. This includes verifying the purpose of the evaluation with the requestor. Although it might seem that this is an unnecessary step, oftentimes it is true that the requesting party has not thought through the entire claim or case, and in some situations, the conversation between IME physician and requesting party can shed new light on certain aspects of a claim that the requesting party has not thought about. Additionally, the requesting party may be somewhat new to the IME process; they may be an entry-level claims examiner who has been trained as to

D.W. Martin, *Independent Medical Evaluation*,
https://doi.org/10.1007/978-3-319-71906-1_6

when an IME should be requested, but has little experience in what the process entails or exactly how the information can be useful to them as a claims evaluator.

Clarification of purpose also refers to the importance of confirming the mechanical aspects of the appointment including those informational items such as time, date, and location of appointment. It also includes a verification and acknowledgment of the business parameters that are germane to the process such as scheduling rules, no-show issues, payment, report deadlines, and other items that were previously discussed in Chapter 4.

It is also at this time that an understanding of the report standard be confirmed. In most situations, there is no "set" format that a report must follow, and if the requesting party is new to the IME examiner, it may be helpful to send an example report and ask if the format is acceptable. In other jurisdictions, such as some state workers' compensation systems, the IME report must follow a rather rigid format. Of course, in this situation, there is little room for creativity with the report document; however the learned IME physician often devises unique ways of staying within the format requirements but also implementing changes that not only adds to the value of the information contained within the report but also indicates to the requesting party that special attention has been paid to their claim. Examples of these types of changes include the use of color, varying the font on subheadings, offsetting of paragraphs, and the use of pictures or drawings.

It is useful during this clarification phase to also understand whether the purpose of the examination is for employability or disability determination. IME reports tend to be a bit different depending upon the focus. In an employability determination, the usual vein of discussion and decision-making is oriented toward what the individual being examined CAN do, whereas in a disability determination, attention is typically turned toward what the individual CANNOT do.

The IME physician must also understand what laws govern the examination. There may be statutes that cover who can and cannot be in the examination room, for example. Other laws may allow or disallow recording, either audio or video. There may be requirements as to how quickly the report must be completed and also who can and cannot receive the report document.

At this juncture, it is also a good idea to have an understanding of who the reader of your report will be (there may be a whole host of individuals) and more importantly what level of expertise the reader has. It is important to understand that some readers will have little if any medical background, and for those readers, staying away from medical terminology or providing a glossary is helpful. There is obviously a difference between writing a Social Security Comprehensive Examination report and an IME report on an individual who is a claimant in a professional liability (malpractice) action.

One way to think about the clarification of purpose is to also remember that the report should be considered a legal document that will be available in perpetuity, unless the rules or statutes that govern the circumstance dictate otherwise. Careful preparation by the IME physician will help avoid uncomfortable issues that might come up in the future. For example, you might be surprised in a deposition that an opposing attorney has brought with them a report of yours from 10 years ago and that your style or methods are not the same as what they are now. While it is certainly acceptable for IME physicians to be on a path of continuous quality improvement, they should also be aware and prepared for these sorts of things, and being consistent in the approach in clarifying the purpose of the IME will go a long way to ensure that you will not have to worry about potential inconsistencies.

Complete Preparation

Preparation for the IME begins with a comprehensive review of all pertinent records. These include not only the medical records but also any nonmedical records when deemed appropriate and relevant to the questions that need to be answered.

In Chapter 5, we discussed how a review of the medical records can set the stage for the IME physician in so far as they give the background of the medical issues at hand and will provide important details regarding the claimant and their status. A review of records will also lead the IME physician to focus upon certain critical areas and help them to develop questions that will be asked during the history-taking part of the IME.

The IME physician will be asked to look at laboratory data. It must be emphasized that the IME physician should be familiar with various laboratory reports and what they mean. Reference ranges that are specific to certain blood tests, for example, may be different from laboratory to the next. The sensitivity and specificity of each laboratory test, while not listed within the context of the laboratory report, is often a sticking point in many claims, and the IME physician, if dealing with these issues, should have a good understanding of the biostatistics that are involved.

Frequently, radiographic reports will be a part of the medical record to review. It is important that the IME physician obtain the studies themselves, which is becoming easier in the digital age of radiology where CT, MRI, and plain film X-rays can be shared on computer systems or copied onto CD or flash drive. Radiologists can make mistakes. Also, especially in reviewing MRI scans, there is quite a variation in radiology terminology from one radiologist to the next. One radiologist's disc "bulge" may be the other's disc "herniation." Terms such as "encroachment," "stenosis," "impingement," "insult," "narrowing," "crowding," "constriction," and "compression" are used to describe exiting nerve root anatomy, but what do they really mean?

But, it is also important that the IME physician not make judgments or comments that lie outside their level of expertise. Some non-radiologist and nonsurgical physicians (like me) were fortunate and had excellent tutelage and time in formal residency to feel very comfortable in reviewing MRIs. But, others may not have had the same opportunities and must then only rely upon the interpretation of the studies that have been provided.

In Chapter 5, the issue of surveillance and investigative reports as well as other nonmedical records was touched upon. The general guiding principle should be that the medical information should drive the medical opinions. Other information, such as private investigation video and attendance or discipline records, can certainly give the IME physician a flavor of the dynamics of a claim, but this information should never be used as a stand-alone basis for a medical determination.

Complete preparation also demands of the IME physician a degree of thought regarding just exactly how the examination is going to occur. Since the IME evaluation is very different than the traditional physician-patient encounter, the IME physician when starting out may feel uneasy about the closing of the encounter when there is no discussion about the diagnosis or treatment plan. It is helpful for the IME physician to develop a script of sorts to follow. Many IME physicians have written templates that they use for history taking, and indeed there are many of these that are available commercially. Other IME physicians have developed their own templates. Others prefer to write questions during the review of records prior to the examination so that they remember to ask those questions during the evaluation itself. Regardless, it is recommended that some format be followed.

Such is also the case with a script for the physical examination. When the IME physician is to determine an impairment rating, templates for the examination are valuable because they will list the specific examination technique and often times also how it is to be done. For example, when measuring range of motion of the shoulder, the *AMA Guides to the Evaluation of Permanent Impairment* demands that six values across three planes of motion be measured with a goniometer a minimum of three different times and in certain anatomical positions. Instead of the IME physician having to recall this type of detail, scripts that can be followed and filled in when the steps are completed can be extremely helpful and ensure that no important part of the examination has been forgotten. It is indeed a bit embarrassing to think that you have completed all the appropriate ROM and other musculoskeletal tests and then find out when you are sitting down and calculating the impairment rating that a certain ROM has been missed!

It is also helpful for the IME physician to think about how they will conclude the examination. Since it may seem odd to not have a discussion with the examinee about their diagnosis and what you would recommend for treatment, it is incumbent upon the IME physician to conclude the evaluation so that both the doctor and the claimant come away with an understanding of the role the IME physician plays while also being comprehensive about the process. One helpful method is to, at the conclusion of the examination, use verbiage such as this:

> "Mrs. X, thank you for your being here today and for telling me about your situation. I have completed my evaluation. I want to make sure that I have not forgotten anything that is important. Is there anything else that you think that we have not covered or gone over today that you believe is important to tell me about?"

Or

> "Thank you, Mr. Y, for your being here and being so cooperative with my evaluation today. I believe that I have covered everything I need to, but no one is perfect and I want to make sure that I have a good understanding of all of your concerns and any details that I might have missed. Is there any other information or details that I have not covered or may have left out that you would like to talk to me about?"

Using these types of open-ended questions and approaches does two things: it allows the IME physician a palatable way to conclude the examination without feeling awkward, and it allows the examinee the opportunity to openly discuss any issue that the IME physician may have omitted or for which the examinee wishes to further explain.

The last issue regarding complete preparation is to discuss the importance of the examinee's reading and signing of an informed consent. The notice of informed consent for IME is important because it establishes the ground rules for the performance of the service and also provides the opportunity for the examinee to understand the rationale for the IME and what the IME provider can and cannot do.

IME informed consents should include an acknowledgment that the examinee understands that there will be no doctor-patient relationship established and that there will not be a discussion regarding diagnoses nor any recommendations for treatment. The document should also indicate that the examinee is consenting to having their history taken and that an examination will occur. The consent form should be clear in stating that the IME physician is independent and that any opinions developed are given irrespective of anyone else involved in the claim (a third-party evaluation). The document should also include a statement that there is an understanding that the results of the evaluation (the report) will only be given to the requesting party (unless there is a jurisdictional rule that requires something else).

It is recommended that appropriate time be spent on this process and that the IME physician be available to provide further answers to questions or clarify points that are not well understood. It is my observation that in reality, very little (if any) time is actually spent on this important step in the IME physician's office. Unfortunately, all too often the examinee signs the form without reading it "just because" they are used to signing a bevy of other forms that they have previously encountered with other health-care encounters or signs it without understanding what it says. Most IME physicians have encountered situations where the examinee has supposedly read and signed the IME consent only to then have the examinee ask the physician about what they recommend next for their condition or ask how they could get a copy of the report. Of course, this sort of situation mandates that the physician pause and return to the consent that the examinee had just signed and re-review with the examinee the specifics of the form so that no further misunderstanding (or non-understanding) situations will hopefully occur.

An example of an informed consent for IME is included at the end of this chapter. This form can be used and modified at your discretion and can be amended to your specific circumstance and applicable rules for your jurisdiction.

A question sometimes arises as to what the IME physician should do if the examinee refuses to sign the notice of informed consent. First, the physician should attempt to explore with the examinee the reason. Often, the hesitancy in signing the form is based upon the examinee not understanding what the IME is intended to accomplish or based upon fear and in some cases advice that the examinee "should not sign anything" in the context of the claim process. Often, and with careful explanation, the IME physician can provide additional explanations as to what is exactly going to happen. With that added information and assurance, most examinees are then willing to sign the form and proceed with the examination.

In some cases, though, the examinee refuses to sign the document. In some cases, they have been instructed to do so by their attorney, and in other cases they do not sign because they are personally opposed to some of the general precepts that surround IME provision. While examinees certainly have the right to NOT being examined, there may be consequences of this decision within the parameters of the benefit system to which they have made a claim. Indeed, most jurisdictions provide for cessation of paid benefits and even claim closure if a requesting party's IME is refused based upon these grounds.

The IME physician is best served by not pursuing with the evaluation in cases where the consent is not signed. Although some IME physicians may be tempted to go on with the evaluation if verbal consent is obtained (without a signature), it is thought that the best practice is to obtain a written consent. There are examples cited when IME physicians elect to conduct the examination when the examinee refuses to sign the consent; many times, the report will indicate the reason for not signing, but it is my perspective that the IME physician assumes significant risk if they elect to do so and I generally recommend against this practice.

Content

Content refers to the actual process of conducting the proper history and physical examination.

As is typically the case with any medical encounter, the history is taken first. Although most physicians are reasonably well trained in their formal education in history taking, several points need to be emphasized.

The timing and circumstances of the onset of symptoms are critical to understand. The IME physician should spend a substantial amount of time on this during the history. If there is a traumatic event, the location and position of the body and any and all outside external forces and conditions should be explored and well understood. The severity of the trauma should be explored, not just in terms of the examinee's perception but what occurred after the specific event in question. As an example, much more detail should be obtained with respect to a slip and fall injury other than just asking when it happened and what the person slipped on. Mechanics of what was the person doing when the slip happened (walking, running, sliding, etc.); whether they were carrying anything when they fell; whether they slipped forward, backward, or sideways; and what they impacted on the way down (something other than the ground?) should be explored. Understanding the terrain of the ground (slippery, unsteady, uneven) can be very important just as it is important to determine if the person tried to break their fall (fall on an outstretched hand, impacted their knees before their torso, etc.). The severity of the fall can be estimated by asking about what happened immediately after the fall. Did the person immediately get back up? Did they need to have help in getting back up? Did they have to sit there and call for help? Finally, asking about whether the fall was witnessed by anyone is important to know as the witness can help in verifying the accuracy and validity of the historical information given by the examinee.

In addressing "cumulative trauma" claims or other exposures, a focus of attention should be on the activities that are being claimed to have caused the medical problem. Specific information regarding the length of time on the job, hours spent per day with a task, whether the person rotates to other activities, and breaks are crucial factors to consider. Also, important to ask about are whether there are any other co-workers who are known to have similar problems, whether there have been any changes to the job tasks over time to minimize (or in some cases worsen) the exposures, or whether any machinery being worked with has changed or has had breakdown or maintenance issues.

A unique factor in the IME history is that the IME physician can review the medical record with the examinee. The physician should discuss with the examinee important findings from physical or mental health exams prior and explore the examinee's understanding of their significance. Such is also the case with any results from prior tests. It can be surprising to some IME physicians regarding how misinformed the examinees sometimes are with these important items. Asking the examinee about their spinal MRI and reports of physical examination from a treating doctor may, for example, yield the following dialogue:

IME physician: "I see that Dr. M saw you and ordered an MRI of your low back on January 21, 2008, is that correct?"

Examinee: "Yes, that's right."

IME physician: "Did he explain to you why he wanted to do that?"

Examinee: "He told me he wanted to see the herniated disc he saw on my regular X-ray."

IME physician: "Were you having any leg pain or numbness at that time?"

Examinee: "No, I don't think I have ever had any leg problems with this."

IME physician: "Then I see after your MRI scan that Dr. M sent you for an epidural injection."

Examinee: "Yes, that's correct."

IME physician: "Did Dr. M tell you what he was trying to help with that?"

Examinee: "Yes, he wanted to try to avoid sending me for back surgery."

This dialogue is not necessarily uncommon. What if the MRI in question here showed a disc bulging at L 4–5 without nerve involvement in a person of 55 years of age? As you can see, the example sheds substantial light on a host of possibilities that could be a problem. The examinee may not have understood the treating physician at all. Looking at the treating physician record will tell the IME physician whether the events recounted by the examinee where accurate. But, the examinee could be correct, and in that case what the IME physician would be interested in is whether the treating physician had actually made an incorrect diagnosis or whether there was a movement down a road of treatment not supported by evidence-based medicine.

The historical trend of symptoms should also be explored and noted. As with any medical condition, attention should be paid to those activities or factors that alleviate and aggravate symptoms. A discussion should occur, using the prior medical records as a backdrop, regarding what medical treatments have been helpful and which have not. While addressing treatment outcomes, it is also very important to understand the examinee's compliance with the recommended treatment plans. If there is information within the record that shows that compliance was an issue, the subject should be explored with the examinee in an attempt to understand the reasons as to why it was a problem.

If the usual progression or resolution of symptoms for a diagnosed condition does not follow what is typical for a given condition, the IME physician should try to figure out why. Is there a misdiagnosed condition? Is there an alternative explanation for the continued or worsening symptoms in the face of a condition that typically improves with time and minor medical involvement? Such possibilities that should be explored by the IME physician include the likelihood of medically unexplained symptoms (MUPS) which can be part and parcel of what is now called somatic symptom disorder. While the issue of somatic symptom disorder and its caveats far exceed the focus of this book, the possibility of this disorder will lead the IME physician to explore such important historical items as adverse childhood experiences; prior spousal, sexual, or other forms of abuse; prior claim behavior; and the context within which a claim has been made.

Many IME physicians administer history questionnaires to their examinees. The benefit of this approach is that it tends to save the physician time in that it can serve as a baseline template for a medical history. Drawbacks to having a questionnaire completed include that there is no predictability as to how long it will take the examinee to complete and thus may throw off the physician's schedule and the fact that handwriting can be a problem to decipher. Additional concerns are how the IME physician is going to approach forms that are incomplete. In some cases, a nondisclosure of information on a questionnaire can be rooted in embarrassing information that the examinee does not want to disclose and in other cases may be intentional because sharing that information might be perceived as being detrimental to their claim.

Some IME physicians have elected to send out history questionnaires to the examinee prior to the IME appointment to avoid these issues. However, one concern with this protocol is that you are not sure if the examinee is the one completing the questionnaire. In some cases, it may be the examinee's attorney who has completed it. I am aware that many IME physicians consider a history questionnaire to be an invaluable part of their examination process. In my opinion, I have found that not to be the case.

Having experimented with a variety of history questionnaires over my career, I have determined that in my practice, I am more efficient if I develop a set list of specific questions based upon the records that I have reviewed and then can explore more details if necessary once those questions are answered. Thus, I do not use questionnaires personally, although many do. My suggestion is to simply do what works best for you. If you do decide to use history questionnaires, there are a plethora of available options that are easily obtainable by a simple web search.

A helpful tool that can be an integral part of the history however is the utilization of a symptom drawing. I prefer to not use the term "pain drawing" even though it may be more common to do so, because a symptom drawing can provide much more useful information. With a symptom drawing, the examinee is asked to notate the anatomical location of certain symptoms with letter designations on a typical stick person outline drawing that is common to most medical professionals. As opposed to using x's, o's, dashes, or some other designation, use of letters that stand for certain symptoms can be more to the point and also allow for overlap of symptoms in certain areas. As it is commonly stated, "a picture paints a thousand words," and an understanding of the examinee's symptoms is often improved when using these diagrams as opposed to simply recording a narrative. Examples of symptom drawings are numerous, but I have included one that I prefer at the end of this chapter and it can be incorporated into your IME protocols at your discretion.

Once the history is obtained, the physical or mental examination is completed.

I consider the physical exam to begin the moment that I begin observing the examinee. This includes looking out my window and watching them walk into the clinic and down the hallway. Seasoned IME examiners, when possible, derive considerable benefit to having their office windows turned toward their office parking areas and offices that provide sight lines down hallways. You will be surprised many times an examinee's gait patterns and behaviors can change in these various areas. You may also be surprised as to how canes and other assistive walking devices are forgotten in exam rooms, thrown into automobile trunks after at the end of appointments, etc. It is also useful to observe the interaction of the examinee with individual's other than you as the examiner. Do they treat everyone the same? Do they put on a different tone and demeanor for you as the examiner only to show something completely different to your office staff? These types of differences can shed significant light upon the claim behavior of the examinee and validity of their complaints.

Prior to the examination, it is important to review with the examinee that they should refrain from doing anything that might cause undue harm or discomfort with any physical exam maneuver or activity. This is necessary because the IME physician is in an atypical situation regarding the exercise of their profession as there is no physician-patient relationship and therefor the conditions that cover professional activity, including that of professional liability, are different. If an "injury" occurs during the examination, usually professional liability and any insurance coverage that the IME physician may have in their more traditional practice encounters would not apply. Rather, allegations of injury during an IME would typically arise under the auspices of either a general liability situation or perhaps even under a charge of assault and battery. If such a report is made, it should be documented in the IME report so that the details of the complaint are known.

If the examinee must disrobe for the examination, it is preferable to wait to do this until after the history is complete. The IME physician should ensure that there is adequate privacy and dignity by providing suitable attire for the examination such as a gown, shorts, tank top, or other forms of draping. It is also important to have a chaperone when appropriate as again, we are not dealing with a typical medical encounter but one that is outside those constraints, and the IME physician should take steps necessary to avoid any potential issues with possible claims of inappropriate examinee contact. When a chaperone is used, it should be documented in the report.

Many IME physicians have established a practice of using a chaperone for the entire IME process, including the history and the physical examination. This methodology has benefit in that the chaperone can not only serve as a witness to the events if there were ever to be a challenge to certain portions of the evaluation process, but they may also serve other functions as scribe for history taking and also provide assistance for certain portions of the examination. Obviously, the chaperone should be the same sex as the examinee.

Just as it was discussed that templates and forms can be helpful for the history, so too can it be helpful for the physical examination. Many IME physicians use preprinted forms that are organ specific; in other words, they may use physical exam worksheets for the upper extremity, spine, vision, and hearing, for example. Such worksheets can facilitate the recording of certain observations and measurements and often will ensure a more complete exam by prompting recollection of certain physical examination tests that might otherwise be forgotten. Additionally, when an examination is being done for purposes of determining an impairment rating, worksheets can be useful as they direct the IME physician on how and how often a particular exam or test must be done. For example, when measuring the range of motion of the lumbar spine with a two-inclinometer technique, worksheets can have designated spaces to record the upper and lower inclinometer readings for flexion, extension, and lateral flexion and also a place to record the supine straight leg raising angle for each leg which is used as a validity determinant.

In the course of providing the examination, the components of an IME which are not typically performed in the context of a treating provider exam but which take on more significance and importance are the repeating of measurements such as range of motion of joints and also strength of certain muscle groups. Usually, impairment rating and other disability systems require a minimum of three trials to establish consistency and validity of the measurement, with the ability to repeat another three trials for a maximum of six in order to establish maximum effort of the examinee.

Also, the examination will typically involve the performance and recording of the so-called "nonorganic" physical findings. Nonorganic findings are physical findings that do not have a direct anatomical cause and are distinct from physical findings of organic pathology. They were first identified in 1980 by Gordon Waddell, the father of the most famous of these signs, the "Waddell Signs," used in the evaluation of low back pain. Although these findings were initially described in patients with low back pain, they may be adapted to patients with neck pain—such as those injured in a car crash. According to Waddell, nonorganic findings "provide a simple and rapid screen to help identify the few patients who require more detailed evaluation." The observation of nonorganic signs is one aspect of the physical examination and is independent of the anatomic and physiological components.

It cannot be underscored enough that the IME physician be extremely well versed in their knowledge of what physical examination techniques are required to be done and what must be recorded, especially if an impairment rating determination is to be completed. For example, knowing that in a complex regional pain syndrome evaluation the *AMA Guides to the Evaluation of Permanent Impairment, Sixth Edition*, requires observation and measurement of such items as skin color, texture, hair distribution, and temperature is critical because the impairment rating numerical calculation hinges upon the number of these items found at the time of the examination. As yet another example, when performing an impairment rating evaluation on an examinee who has had a total knee replacement, it is required that the physician measure and record knee alignment and also any degree of medial-lateral instability. These two examples illustrate uncommon physical examination observations and measurements when a physician is in a treating capacity, but for which are an absolute necessity for an IME physician to know and understand.

Digital photographs can be invaluable to include within the context of the physical examination and, in many cases, can be of extreme help when added to the IME report. Photographs can help document scars from insults such as burn injuries and surgical complications as well as skin grafts and can provide a visual record of the problem that a narrative may not necessarily be able to do with the same level of comprehensiveness. Photographs can also be helpful when there are claims by the examinee of extremity swelling or discoloration. But, the IME physician must be aware that these photographs can be just as important in documenting the nonexistence of these examinee reports as they are helpful when they indeed exist. Such is the case when an examinee makes a claim of swelling in an extremity injury claim but for which the examiner cannot tell the difference between the injured side and the non-injured opposite arm or leg.

Lastly, many IME physicians elect to utilize computerized or machine-based range of motion or strength evaluations. The advantages of this approach are that this typically eliminates intra-rater reliability issues where the same examiner might exhibit some variability when they use a goniometer, for example. Another advantage is that subtle strength losses may be identified with these devices that provide a degree of precision greater than the standard 5 grade scale manual muscle test that is looked upon as a standard. Caution should be given when deciding to introduce these devices into the examination process as they are only as good as the individual who has set them up for use. Also, many examinees have strong fear avoidance to being tested in the manner by a machine, and reproducibility and maximum effort are frequently not achieved. These computerized or digital devices also tend to be quite expensive, so the IME physician should make an informed decision about their utility based upon a level of confidence and risk-benefit analysis taking into consideration all of the issues in a purchase and use decision.

Like what was previously discussed with respect to the conclusion of taking the history, the IME physician should have a standard approach to concluding the examination. As the physical examination is typically the final part of the IME encounter with the physician, it is prudent to ask the examinee how they are doing and whether there is anything else that they would like the doctor to check. A typical ending statement by the IME physician may be something like this:

> "Mr. Y, I am finished with my examination and I want to thank you for being cooperative regarding that with me today. Now that I am done with my physical examination, I want to make sure that you are doing okay and that you are not experiencing any troubles. Are you doing fine? Great. Lastly, with all of my evaluations, I always want to make sure that I have not forgotten anything or skipped over anything that you think is important. Is there anything that you would like me to examine and document that I have not done so far? Is there anything else that you want to tell me? Okay, thank you again."

Communication

Although we will review in detail within Chapter 9 the authoring and creation of the IME report, an integral part of communication and an exercise that has become an important part of the IME process is to ask the examinee to complete an exit interview or satisfaction survey after the examination but before they leave the office. The best way to accomplish this is to discuss the survey with the examinee and give it to them to complete once the physical examination is completed and before they leave the examination room. The easiest method to accomplish this is for the IME physician to have this survey with them and to review the importance of its completion immediately once the examination is concluded as there is a much better completion rate when the examinee knows that it must be filled out before they can go. Although it does not necessarily insure its completion, if the IME physician explains that the survey is a standard form that is done with an eye toward continuous quality improvement, most examinees are perfectly happy to comply with the task to have the form completed.

Such satisfaction surveys can ask questions regarding the adequacy and clarity of communication from the IME physician's office about directions to the office, the quality of the interaction with the office staff, and the physical appearance of the office itself. However, these satisfaction surveys can provide a quite different function for the IME physician, that being that it serves as a record against which future accusations that the IME was not comprehensive can be measured or can provide a defense against claims that "the doctor hurt me" during the exam. Thus, these exit interviews or surveys can ask questions such as whether the examinee felt the exam was comprehensive, whether any part of the examination caused pain, or whether enough time was spent by the IME physician. Finally, an overall rating regarding the examinee experience can be obtained and can be used in any promotional items that the IME physician may elect to use. An example of an exit interview or satisfaction survey is included at the end of this chapter which may be adapted for use in your IME practice.

Appendix 1: Notice of Informed Consent for Independent Medical Evaluation

This is to verify that I am to undergo a medical evaluation related to my claim of injury, illness, impairment or disability conducted by Any Doctor MD on ____________________(date).

I understand that this evaluation is to include my giving information about myself and my personal circumstance as well as my health.

I understand that there is also to be a physical examination, which may be performed on any relevant part of my body, and that I may be asked to undergo certain tests and x-rays. I acknowledge that no audio or video recording will occur during this examination.

I understand that an Independent Medical Evaluation (IME), by definition, means that no doctor-patient relationship has or can be established and that Dr. Doctor cannot be involved in the care of my injury or illness.

I understand that within the context of an IME, results of this evaluation cannot be given to me, and that any report(s) generated by this evaluation can be given only to the party requesting the examination and that if I or my representative desire a copy of any report(s) generated, that the inquiry be directed to the party requesting the examination.

I understand that the purpose of this examination is to obtain an independent, third party opinion, that all of the findings will be neutral and that the evaluator has no role in the claims decision process or results thereof.

(Signed) ________________________________

(Date) ___________________________

Appendix 2: Symptom Drawing Example

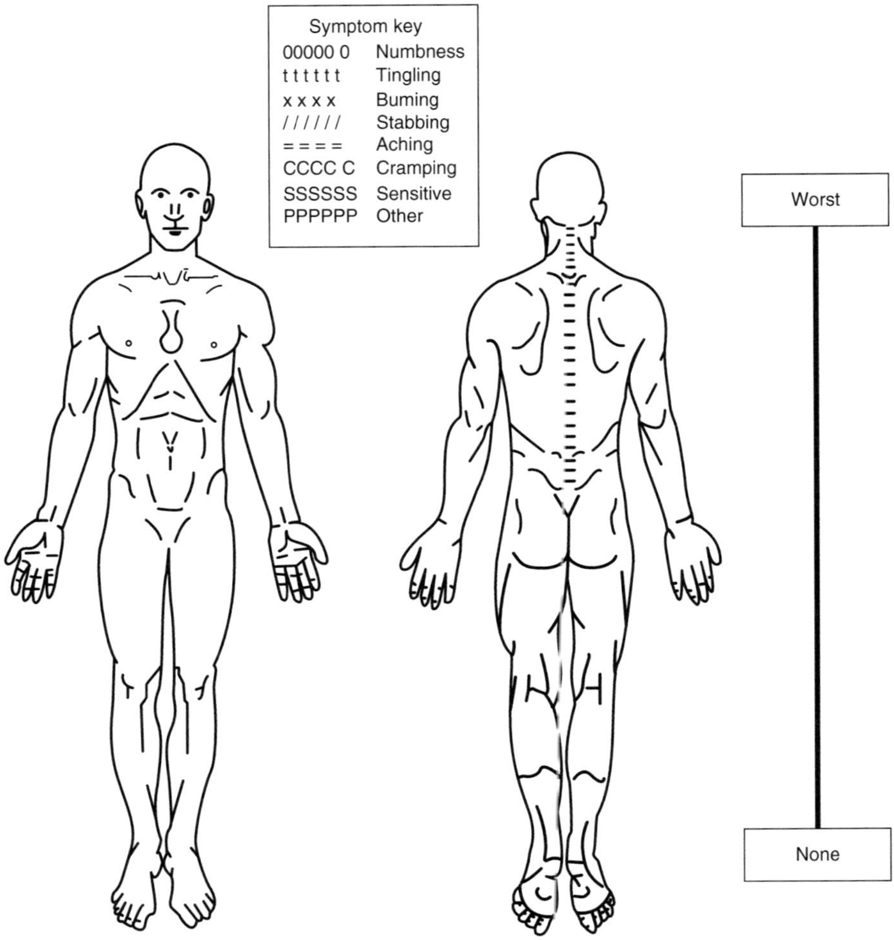

Appendix 3: Exit Interview Example

IME Exit Survey

Thank you for your appointment today for your independent medical examination. So that we can strive to continually improve upon our service, we ask that you complete this short survey about your experience today. Please circle the answers.

1. In general, my overall impression with my evaluation was:
   Excellent Good Average Below average Poor

2. I felt that the evaluation was comprehensive.
   Yes No

3. I thought the doctor listened to my concerns:
   Yes No

4. I felt that there was enough time given to this evaluation:
   Yes No

5. Did you experience any pain or injury from the examination?
   Yes No

   If yes, please describe: ______________________________

6. Do you have any other comments you would like to share?

   ____
   ____
   ____

Thank you for completing this survey

______________________ ______________________

Name Date

Bibliography

1. Freeman G. Tips for writing reports. Conference proceedings of the AADEP Comprehensive Training Course, Chicago, 31 March 1998. Chicago: American Academy of Disability Evaluating Physicians.
2. Martin D. The independent medical examination. Conference proceedings of the 102nd American occupational health conference, Denver, Colorado, 24 April 2017. Chicago: American College of Occupational and Environmental Medicine.
3. Nierenberg C, Brigham C, Direnfield L, Burket C. Standards for independent medical examinations. Guides Newsletter; Nov/Dec 2005.

7 Be Prepared!: Things You May Not Have Thought About

"Be Prepared" is the motto of the Boy Scouts of America. As an Eagle Scout and one who is still quite involved as an adult leader and volunteer, there is no better motto that is more appropriate to follow for the IME physician. IMEs are different. The whole process might be considered an outlier by your colleagues, and organized or mainstream medicine may consider them so far off the radar screen that the mere mention of them casts raised eyebrows and even cynicism.

They are unique to pretty much everything else that a physician could elect to do with their professional practices. With nearly 25 years of experience, I would like to touch on a few things that you may not have thought about and some suggestions to keep you from worrying about them.

What Happens When They Ask You to Treat?

Even though you have painstakingly gone through the notice of informed consent document that clearly states that they are acknowledging that the IME does not establish a doctor-patient relationship, you will still probably encounter a situation where an examinee asks if they can have you treat their problem or whether they can see you again for some other reason. When asked, I recommend that you take a time-out during the history or physical examination and get out the notice of informed consent and go over it with them again. It is best to explain also verbally that by affixing their signature to the consent, they have notarized that this must be the case if they were to rescind the consent that the IME would have to be terminated and that no report could be generated. Of course, it is best to do this in a kind and matter-of-fact matter to avoid any disdain from the examinee.

D.W. Martin, *Independent Medical Evaluation*,
https://doi.org/10.1007/978-3-319-71906-1_7

What Happens When They Want the Entire Family in the Room?

The issue of who is in the examination room and who is not is always an issue. As I have previously stated, it is best to limit the examination to only the examinee themselves, with the exception being when evaluating a case of neuropsychological impairment from head trauma or other cognitive dysfunction from other illnesses. In these cases it is sometimes helpful to have the spouse or one other close family member in the room to provide information on the history that the examinee may not be able to answer.

But, you will be faced with situations when entire families may want to be present, sometimes children. Previously, we addressed the importance of sending out a confirmation letter within which it should be explained that the examinee should not bring other people with them to the examination because of the fact that the IME physician cannot accommodate for this. Despite this, if the examinee does have, for example, three children with her, you will have to make a decision on whether to continue with the IME or not. In most of these situations, I would strongly suggest not to proceed.

Another difficulty is when the examinee or their representative demands that an observer be present for the evaluation. This is a difficult situation for the IME physician in that this may be a person who is not a family member who can add to the history. It has been shown that the presence of an observer during a third-party evaluation will actually compromise the credibility of the evaluation [1, 2]. Many IME physicians have used the scientific research on this subject successfully to bar observers from the exam room.

What Happens When They Try to Record You?

You will eventually run into a situation where an examinee will want to record you with a tape device or as is more commonly the case now with one of the various smartphones that have recording capabilities. Smartphones (and other telephones for that matter) can also be left on for the entire course of the examination and linked to software that will save the entire contents in a file. Rarely will you encounter an examinee who wishes to videotape the encounter, because most do not have the proper equipment to do so.

It is recommended to not allow such recording. Some IME physicians elect to place a statement within the notice of informed consent that covers this, which can be a very good idea if the examinee attempts to record the evaluation without the knowledge of the physician.

You may ask why allowing a recording is a bad practice. The reason is that such recordings serve no real purpose other than as an attempt to discredit the IME physician's comprehensiveness about either the history or the physical exam or both. Tapes can be edited, and even though the IME physician may be completely thorough in their approach and processes, an altered tape could be shown that might portray just the opposite. Additionally, it has been shown that recording such an encounter can invalidate the history, even subconsciously, because the examinee has a tendency to not be as forthcoming in answering questions when they know that they have the potential to have their answers critiqued in the future.

When an examinee either asks or is found to be recording during the examination, the IME physician should stop and review the policy (and notice of informed consent if it includes such a statement) and ask that the tape device or smartphone be shut off before pursing with the remainder of the evaluation. This is an event or occurrence that should also be recorded in the IME written report, so that the attempt is documented for the future. While it may not be possible (or legal) to attempt to confiscate the equipment or the tape, the IME physician does have an obligation to point out that their policy of non-recording has been breached. If the examinee refuses to stop the recording, then it is suggested that the IME be terminated.

There are many interesting stories that I have heard about some of my colleagues about creative ways that taping and recording have been handled. One such story involved an IME examiner who discovered that he was being taped right after the completion of the history and right before they started with the examination, noting that the examinee had hidden a tape recorder under their leg while sitting on the examination room table, only to have it fall to the floor when the exam began. Instead of the physician terminating the exam, they elected to pick up the recorder and speak loudly right into it, saying "Oh My God!!!" and then subsequently completing the remainder of the examination in total silence, using hand gestures and written instructions to complete the physical examination.

You may be in a rare jurisdiction where the recording of an IME is allowed under law. If you find yourself in this situation, you have a decision to make. Either you can elect to conduct the examination or not. If you elect to do so and it is going to be taped or recorded, a strong recommendation is to have someone that you have selected to also record it at the same time. In this manner, you can ensure that the party who is recording you will not attempt to edit or cut out certain portions of the recording.

What Happens When They Have "Mad at the World Syndrome"?

You will encounter examinees who do not want to be present for your IME. In some cases, IMEs have been agreed upon by two opposing parties in a legal case or have been scheduled by an opposing party whom the examinee distrusts or simply has ill will against. So too will you have examinees who have what I call "mad at the world syndrome" who seemingly have a poor attitude about everything and treat everyone in your clinic poorly.

Clearly, if you encounter an examinee that is abusive or threatening to either you or your staff, the encounter should be stopped immediately, and the requesting party should be notified as soon as possible.

Most examinees, however, are not like this. While they may have poor demeanors, rarely are there problems. There are some strategies that the IME physician can employ to mitigate these types of situations.

No individual typically likes to make a scene in front of a crowd. Thus, it is often suggested that IMEs be conducted in locations where there are many other patients or staff that will be around.

Also, it is helpful to train your staff to be overly nice. This helps if you have an examinee that is angry or feels victimized. As a matter of fact, since your staff really has no authoritative role in your IME or your opinions, you can train your staff to provide unconditional positive regard in their encounters with the examinee. Such an encounter with the receptionist and nursing staff prior to seeing the IME doctor might go something like this:

Examinee at the receptionist window: "Someone wants me to see this doctor here."

Receptionist: "Hi there. You must be Mr. Pissdoff. I am really glad you made it to our clinic today and am so happy you were early for your appointment! I will go get the nurse who will show you to the exam room and have you complete some basic paperwork."

Nurse: "Hello Mr. Pissdoff. I am the doctor's nurse. I am going to be your guide today through the exam. If you have any questions, or need anything, you make sure you ask me and I will make it happen."

Examinee: "I don't want to be here. The insurance company made me do this. It's a bunch of bullshit."

Nurse: "Yes, we hear that from a lot of folks. It's too bad, I know. I don't like insurance companies either. But, I will try to get you through this as fast as possible so you can be on your way."

Examinee: "I don't know. I have seen so many doctors I am tired of it! Your doctor probably works for the insurance company."

Nurse: "I am indeed sorry, and I know how frustrating your situation must be. We had several folks in here this week who are in the same boat! But, I think you will like my doctor. He has been doing this a long time and is a pretty nice person. He has been affiliated with the hospital system here for 25 years."

Examinee: "Well, I guess we will see."

In addition to training your staff to be overly nice, successful IME physicians also tend to be pleasant and upbeat. Now, not everyone can be the Smiling Sally all the time, but what does make a difference is to be consistent in your tone, demeanor, and body language with every IME encounter. Another thing that will go a long way to lessen the angst of the examinee is to spend time with them. I cannot tell you how many times I have been told at the end of an IME "you've spent more time with me today than any of my treating doctors combined." If you are thorough and complete with your evaluation, the examinee will have little to be upset with you about.

It is also a good strategy to eliminate interruptions as much as possible. I strongly suggest that you instruct your staff to not interrupt you during an IME unless it is a true emergency. Leave your pager or phone outside the exam room. Being interrupted is a distraction not only to you but also to the examinee and does not promote an outward appearance of professionalism.

Dealing with Threats Either Real or Veiled

Despite the strategies and interventions above, there may come a time when you must deal with a threat from an examinee. If there is danger to you or your staff, there should be protocols in place to deal with the dangerous or threatening patient, which should also apply here. If there is a need to call 911 or security, then it should be done. Obviously, when a direct threat is made, the IME should be terminated and the requesting party should be notified.

I have personally never encountered a direct threat, but I have heard that other colleagues have. I suppose that it is helpful to be a 6′3″ 275 Ib former football player, but even the daintiest of physician should never have to deal with such an issue.

There are times when there may be veiled threats made in advance of the exam. Examinees, family members, or even attorneys have called stating things like "you had better treat me well or I will do something about it" or even "if I have to go to this exam, I'm probably going to go berserk." So, too, have requesting parties or case management nurses called in advance relaying that the examinee may have caused a scene at another physician's office or have had violent past histories. When these things occur, the IME physician has to make a decision of whether to withdraw from the process or continue. If the decision is to continue, which often times happens at the pleading of the requesting party because such behavior of the examinee is well known and has led to other physicians not wanting to get involved, the IME physician can consider a wide range of options. At my disposal, as I am in a hospital system, are employed security officers. I have had them sit in my waiting room. I have also had a sheriff's deputy sit in an adjacent area so that the IME examinee must walk past them to get to their exam room. It is amazing how docile and pleasant examinees that have shown prior aberrant behaviors can be when such a silent but obvious show of authority and force is present.

Be Careful Who You Talk To

Confidentiality regarding the IME process is critical. In all cases the IME physician should discuss details about the evaluation only with the requesting party or to others only if the requesting party has given written permission. While it might be tempting to respond to written requests of other parties, the IME physician cannot do so unless the requesting party wishes him to.

Scrupulous attorneys and others (even health-care providers) may attempt to get information from you or your report by sending what looks like an official request for records that might even contain a written release. However, since the IME report is NOT a medical record in most jurisdictions and instead is considered an attorney work product, such requests and releases are not germane. Don't be fooled by examinees that list you as a "treating source" especially if they have applied for social security, short-term, or long-term disability benefits. You are NOT a treating source and do not have any obligation to divulge information from your IME to these systems. When such requests for information arise, it is best to always contact the requesting party (referral source) to determine how they wish you to respond (or not). In some cases, they will tell you that it is okay to do so, perhaps because the claim has been settled or the issue is no longer relevant. If this is the case, then careful documentation of the date of permission and items that may be disclosed by the IME physician is necessary. It is also incumbent upon the IME physician to make sure that the party requesting the information understands that you had no treating role with the examinee and within what context the interaction occurred. If forms appear that are to be completed by the "attending" or "treating" physician, the IME doctor must decline, because that is not their role.

Care should also be taken by the IME physician that they do not fall into the trap of casual discussion with a family member of the examinee or other parties. Although it might seem humanistic and appropriate to have a conversation about an examinees' medical problem with their son or daughter or other relative, this should never occur. At the same time, any medical details that are known by your staff because of their handling of documents or interaction with the examinee must be held in strictest confidence. It is best to review this with staff members periodically so as to avoid any mishaps or misunderstanding of the importance of this.

Avoid Being Stereotyped

One of the worst things that can happen to an IME physician is to be stereotyped or labeled as either a "defense friendly" or "plaintiff friendly" expert. This is avoidable by making sure that your opinions and perspectives can always be supported by the medical literature. It is just as important to make sure that when situations arise where there is no literature to support a conclusion, that the IME physician state so. While it is certainly appropriate to offer opinions from a medical perspective, it is critical to make sure that those opinions can be traced to their sources.

Nevertheless, and despite the IME physician painstakingly adhering to evidence-based medicine, these types of stereotypes may occur. If you have an examinee or an examinee's representative that communicates with you either prior to the IME or during it that they believe you are biased toward one side or the other, it is good practice to explain why you are not and that your conclusions will be based upon the information garnered during the history and physical examination and that any opinions will be based upon what evidence is available in the medical literature. Addressing these concerns to the examinee at the beginning of the encounter can be quite helpful as it sets a level playing field for all in the room and promotes a sense of true "independence" of the IME physician in that there will not be a reliance upon other physician's opinions. Frequently, it is helpful to explain to the examinee that you are coming to their claim "as someone new who knows nothing about the past."

The successful IME physician will find that they receive referrals from a variety of sources. If you find yourself receiving referrals only from defense or only from plaintiff attorneys, the IME physician should take pause and review the cases they have been involved with, asking the question, "can all of my opinions prior be supported by the evidence based literature?" If the answer is "yes" then fine, but in many situations the IME physician may need a review of exactly how they got to the place of receiving referrals from only one side of the lawsuit spectrum.

Have a Good Answer When You Are Accused of Working "for" Someone

Examinees and their representatives often have a misperception that you as the IME physician are employed by an insurance company or third-party administrator or even law firms. When these situations arise, it is a best practice to explain that your services have been retained to provide an INDEPENDENT assessment of the medical issues at hand and that your opinion is not for sale. Often, I have found it helpful to explain how I am compensated by my hospital system. Although I am not suggesting that every IME physician must go into detail on how they are paid, since I am an employed physician who is paid by the hospital via a relative value unit (RVU) system, it is easy to explain to the examinee and their representatives that I do not even see a statement, nor do I have knowledge of collections, specific charges, or any other items that have to do with the payment or transfer of money from the requesting party to my hospital system who is the entity that collects the bill.

If that is not enough, it can be further helpful to indicate that your opinions and conclusions could be unfavorable to the requesting party. If you have good examples of this, it can be beneficial to explain in general terms (to not breach confidentiality) situations where this has occurred. Such showing of these examples will help establish that you indeed are independent and that you cannot be "bought or sold" with respect to your medical opinions.

Some Attorneys Do Not Play Fair

Despite your great intentions to provide the best IME service possible, there are and will continue to be what I refer to as "bad actors" in the process. In my experience, these "bad actors" are usually attorneys who appear to have taken their advocacy role for their client to a level that is an obstacle to the performance of a quality IME or who are attempting to simply make so much chaos out of a claim situation that the opposing side will yield to their wishes or demands. The unfortunate problem with this is that the IME physician can be made a pawn in a much larger chess game. Here are some real-world examples of this, all of these based upon my experiences:

- The examinee's attorney intentionally tells their client, the examinee, to not appear for a scheduled appointment as a methodology to extend a case into the future or as a showing of their displeasure with the process.
- The examinee's attorney, when becoming aware of their clients' IME appointment, sends a letter to the IME physician along with medical records, as though they are the requesting party when they are not, sometimes in an attempt to obtain information form the IME physician via a report or some other communication. All this does is confuse the office staff and create duplication of the medical records that you are to review.

- The examinee's attorney, after becoming aware of their client's IME appointment and subsequently knowing your clinic protocols, instructs their client to bring along their spouse, four children, and four brothers and sisters, all of whom demand to be in the room during the IME.
- The examinee's attorney intentionally tells their client to show up late in an attempt to show how rigid and uncaring you are in that you will not see them because it is past the time that your clinic establishes for a "no-show."
- The examinee's attorney, knowing your protocol for the exam, tells their client to show up on time, but tells their client not to sign the IME consent. The examinee is instructed to call the attorney to review the form, which is then signed, but it is now 40 minutes past the time of the start of the appointment.
- The examinee has been instructed by their attorney to intentionally take an inordinate amount of time during the history portion of the exam which is a strategy to irritate the IME physician and put them behind schedule.

When these things happen, the IME physician should remain calm and consistent with their approach. There is absolutely nothing wrong with adhering to your clinic policy on time, no show issues, etc., which illustrate why it is so important to have these things in place when the appointment is made and have prior communication with the requesting party and the examinee so that everyone is on the same page.

It is also not a problem if the IME physician runs out of time during the scheduled allotment for the exam. Another examination time can be requested to complete the task. This is especially true when dealing with the last bullet point example listed above.

What to Do When Attempts Are Made to "Limit" Your Examination

There have been attempts, primarily by those in the legal system, to limit the IME physician's ability to obtain a complete history or perform a comprehensive examination. In these situations, there have even been court orders directing the IME physician to not ask about past history, prior treatments, or other injury claims.

These attempts are made primarily to guard the claimant against what some might consider biasing information or in some cases potentially embarrassing or pejorative facts. The problem is that when you limit a physician's ability to investigate all biopsychosocial factors in a claim, the opinion is no longer valid. Can we actually determine cardiac risk if we can't ask about family history? Are we able to determine current mental status and integrative functioning if we cannot analyze baseline educational records?

If you find yourself the subject of one of these "limited" edicts, I strongly suggest that you remove yourself from the situation. My suggestion is based upon what I consider a "line drawn in the sand" with regard to what is reasonable or not. Limiting the ability of any physician the ability to do their job by performing a complete history and physical examination goes against the very nature and philosophy of medicine itself and cannot and should not be tolerated.

A few years ago, the American Academy of Disability Evaluating Physicians (now known as the International Academy of Independent Medical Evaluators) was asked by one of their members to file an amicus brief when the member received a court order to limit his examination on an upcoming examinee [3]. Portions of a letter describing the amicus brief are included at the end of this chapter. It is added here not because of the details of the claim, but because of the reasons and rationale as to why the IME physician must not be encumbered with such limitations.

Protect Yourself (and with the Right Liability Policy)

IME physicians must make sure that they have the proper professional liability policy that will include their performance of these exams. It is important to note that many professional liability policies written for physicians (commonly referred to as "malpractice insurance") will not cover IME services. The reason is that these policies only apply when a doctor-patient relationship exists. As was stated previously, when an examinee files a lawsuit against an IME physician, it is typically not for malpractice, but can include items such as errors and omissions or even product liability.

Some jurisdictions have deemed that physicians who perform IMEs do have limited liability when it comes to malpractice, even when it is has been firmly established that a care relationship does not exist. One such case in Arizona involved a wrongful death case in which an IME physician opined that the examinee did not have a serious back condition and could return to work without restrictions [4]. The examinee's benefits were terminated, and he became addicted to opioids and eventually died of an overdose. The details of the case are as follows:

> In a suit by his family relating to his wrongful death, a jury in Arizona found an IME doctor to be 28.5 percent responsible/negligent in relation to a man's wrongful death.
>
> Attorneys for the doctor appealed in the case called Ritchie v. Krasner, Arizona Court of Appeals, April 21, 2009. As part of the Appeals Court opinion the court stated as follows:
>
> "We…cannot envision a public benefit in encouraging a doctor with specific individualized knowledge not to investigate the symptoms of a cervical [neck] spine injury. We recognize the very real concern that imposing a duty on [the IME doctor] to practice reasonable care under the circumstances might create a chilling effect within the IME community… [H]owever, ethical standards govern physicians, and they likely limit the threatened flood of litigation to a trickle…we do not hold that every IME physician has a duty of care in every situation. In this case, [the IME doctor] was hired to determine the extent of the…work-related injury and make treatment recommendations. By agreeing to do so, he assumed a duty to conform to the legal standard of reasonable conduct in light of the apparent risk. Therefore we hold that the trial court correctly held that [the IME doctor] owed a duty of reasonable care…."

Thus, IME physicians should be aware of all parameters surrounding their need for proper medical liability coverage. When in doubt, ask your current insurance carrier if IMEs are covered. If you are told they are but it is not crystal clear to you that the policy language is proper, ask for a written acknowledgment. If they are not, ask if there is a rider to the policy that can be written. If this is not possible, then explore insurance carriers who write policies specific for IME provision.

Appendix 1: Selected Portions of Letter Sent to AADEP for Their Response

February 11, 2010

RE: James Williams, Jr. vs. Taylor Banks

Dear AADEP:

As a Fellow of this organization, I wanted to make you aware of recent court imposed limitations that have been proposed, with respect to an upcoming Independent Medical Examination of the above named individual within the context of the lawsuit.

Specifically, the court has indicated the following with regards to this evaluation:

1. "The scope of the examination shall only be for the injuries claimed in the subject wreck and not any unrelated injury."
2. "Mr. Williams should not be questioned by the doctor or his staff regarding details of how the wreck occurred, employment, or other areas outside specific questions about his physical injury."
3. "Mr. Williams shall not be required to produce any documentation or diagnostic test results at the examination."
4. "That the examining doctor's testimony shall be limited in scope to plaintiff's injury from the wreck and shall only be within the scope of his professional specialty."

I find that these limitations impossible to meet, and counter to principles that I have been trained in from your organization and also my past experiences in performing these services.

I would ask that your organization respond to this, if possible.

Sincerely,

Dr. XXXXXXX

Appendix 2: Selected Portions of AADEP Amicus Brief Response

Dear Doctor XXXXXXX:

We received your letter of February 11, 2010 notifying us of your difficulties with regards to an upcoming Independent Medical Examination that you have been asked to perform and the reported court limitations regarding your activities in that process.

The American Academy of Disability Evaluating Physicians has taught physicians of a variety of medical disciplines the performance of proper professionalism and methodologies regarding the performance of Independent Medical Examinations for over two decades.

We find that the limitations that have been posed upon you by the court will not allow any reputable Independent Medical Examiner to be able to comply with those court's prescriptions in good conscience. The limitations would hamper the performance of fair and factual medical examination and is patently opposite to the recommendations of the *AMA Guides, Fifth Edition*, and three other relevant articles from the American Medical Association accompanying *Guides Newsletter*.

Independent Medical Examinations must be nonpartisan with no bias in favor of or against a claimant. Denying a claimant his right to dispute in his own words what he may disagree with is unfair to him. That is why oral history taking must be allowed. The past history of relevant medical problems might have significant pertinence to the current injury, and a prohibition of seeking this data is unfair to the defense. Testimony regarding a past history of similar medical problems is thus absolutely necessary.

We also are aware that other sister organizations to us have weighed in on this topic. One such organization is the American Academy of Orthopedic Surgeons, who has a Physician Statement related to the duties of expert witness testimony. In the first paragraph of this document, it indicates: "By providing testimony that is fair and accurate, an expert witness can contribute to a just outcome in a lawsuit. Testimony that is unfair or inaccurate has negative ramifications beyond the case at hand. Unfair or inaccurate testimony discredits the orthopedic profession and is often cited as a contributing factor to the current professional liability crisis."

While we can understand that the examination should be focused upon the injuries that are involved in a specific wreck at hand, there may be antecedent injuries or injuries of similar areas of the body that have occurred in the past, which would make it impossible to follow this prescription. For example, if a patient has a knee injury in the current accident, but had a history of a knee arthroscopy or previous knee injury - on both that side or on the other side - an examination would be important to understand the nature of the most recent injury. Of course, one would agree that, if the issue was a neck injury and the examination of the big toe would be totally useless, that would not even be attempted in this type of a situation. The decision of whether or not the examination should be made for areas that may be contiguous or in some way medically related to the injury that is under discussion should not be in the purview of the claimant, the claimant's attorney or the court, but should be solely rested with the decision process of the Independent Medical Examiner. Although the examination information may or may not be helpful, it should not be restricted. Who would decide if there is a dispute over which area can or cannot be examined?

With regards to the court order indicating that the examinee should not be questioned by the doctor or his staff regarding details of how the wreck occurred, issues of employment or other area outside specific questions about his physical injury, we note that this would simply be impossible to fulfill as an Independent Medical

Examiner. To limit a medical analyst regarding the determination of accuracy of what happened in the particular wreck, how or how it did not interfere with his employment would be circumspect. It is not possible for a doctor asking questions about the history from an examinee to have a debate on each item of whether or not it fulfills the parameters of the court mandate. It would seem incredulous that the examinee or the examinee's attorney would have authority over what questions are asked by a physician in this context.

Regarding the court's demand that the claimant shall not be required to produce any documentation or diagnostic test results at the examination, this, of course, is something that probably could be adhered to, but one wonders whether it is intended to be more of a roadblock that a reality. Obviously, there are many different ways that an individual could present the diagnostic test documentation or medical record to the Independent Medical Examiner.

With regards to limiting the physician's testimony to the scope of the plaintiff's injury, in reality, that is probably reasonably appropriate. However, we are concerned that this limitation might put the Independent Medical Examiner in such a narrow box that important information regarding disability may not be brought to the forefront, which could be very important and relevant in the individual case.

We would point out that, in the *American Medical Association Guides to the Evaluation of Permanent Impairment, Fifth Edition*, on page 374, under Section 15.1 entitled "Principles of Assessment", the Guides are emphatic in that they say, "The evaluation should include a comprehensive accurate medical history: a review of all pertinent records, a comprehensive description of the individual's current symptoms, and the relationship to daily activities." To limit this to something other than "comprehensive" would seem to be in direct contradistinction to what the *AMA Guides* requires an Independent Medical Examiner to perform.

This long accepted methodology of taking a history by documenting the examinee's own comments and following whatever is required to obtain the proper background information is mandatory for any physician trying to do a proper, accurate and factual Independent Medical Examination. If one relies on the mandates of the Guides and the training that we provide to physicians, the IME physician should be allowed to ask whatever questions they feel are important and relevant to the individual case and claim at hand. To limit the IME physician's inherent ability to obtain a factual history is something that would be very concerning, with regards to these types of evaluations now and even into the future.

We would also point out that there may be instances in which the examinee disagrees with the statements that are made in the record by other physicians. One of the jobs of the IME physician is to identify these discrepancies and try to afford an understanding as to why they exist. It is obviously in the examinee's interest and it is important for the examinee to answer in his own words with regards to these types of discrepancies. It is not fair for the examinee not to be able to describe in their own words what the errors might be, and to try to get a reasonable explanation from their perspective as to why they might exist. This, obviously, cannot occur unless a personal oral history is being obtained from the Independent Medical Examination physician.

In the *Guides Newsletter* of September/October of 2005, in an article written by one of our faculty members and former board members, Dr. Alan Colledge, entitled, "Duties of the Examining Physician", he makes the point that, "The examinee's history should be primarily based upon the individual's own statements rather than secondhand information assuming the individual's statements are reliable. The physician should consider information from all sources, including medical records. Although it is not appropriate to question the individual's integrity, it is appropriate to comment on the individual's credibility. The credibility of patients' representation could be interpreted in light of their consistency across time and in accordance with their objective findings."

In a second article in the *Guides newsletter* of July/August 2006, written by Christopher Brigham, M.D., a Fellow of this Academy and current well known author on the subject, he makes the following comments: "All applicable medical records and other documents that may be helpful in the rating process should be provided. The physician needs to allocate adequate time to performing a thorough evaluation, including obtaining the clinical history, reviewing studies, and performing an appropriate examination."

It is for the above reasons that the American Academy of Disability Evaluating Physicians wishes to file this brief, in this case. We would respectfully ask the court to remove these limitations upon the Independent Medical Examination that is being proposed, in this case. We are very concerned that, if these prohibitions are allowed to stand, they may become universal, which will in essence negate the validity and role that Independent Medical Examinations play in the medicolegal context.

Bibliography

1. Barth R. Observation compromises the credibility of an evaluation. Guides Newsletter; Jul/Aug 2007.
2. Ruttle P. Letter to the editor re: observation compromises the credibility of an evaluation. Guides Newsletter; Jul/Aug 2010.
3. Case No. 2010-CA-000408-OA Jefferson Circuit Court No. 09-CI-005325, Kentucky; 24 March 2011.
4. Appeal from the Superior Court in Maricopa County Cause No. CV 2002-023901; CV 2002-024074, Arizona; 21 April 2009.
5. Brigham C. Erroneous impairment ratings. Guides Newsletter; Jul/Aug 2006.
6. Colledge A. Duties of the examining physician. Guides Newsletter; Sep/Oct 2005.

8 Addressing Common Questions Posed to the IME Examiner

There are several different issues that frequently are needed to be addressed by requesting parties. Several of these will be reviewed below. This is not intended to be an all-encompassing list but is presented to give the Independent Medical Examiner an understanding of the common issues for which IMEs are requested.

Causation

Frequently needed, especially in workers' compensation cases and personal injury claims, is to answer questions regarding causation. Since, in the United States, there are multiple benefit systems in place that cover medical care costs and indemnification based upon what system is claimed, the issue of causation takes more of a center role that in other countries. Assigning responsibility, not only for the costs of medical care regarding any injury or an illness, is important to ferret out, but also is important to assign appropriate compensation regarding permanent problems that exist.

This book is not focused on the issue of biostatistics and epidemiology; however, the IME physician must have a relevant and proper understanding of these principles in order to understand issues of causation analysis.

The legal system has two criteria to establish causation. One is the level of certainty required before an expert medical opinion is legally competent. The second is the issue of basic overall burden of proof, frequently referred to as "preponderance of the evidence." As a result, for a medical opinion about causation to be admitted into the evidence in a legal proceeding, the person offering the opinion needs to attest that he/she holds the opinion with some level of certainty.

There may be some differences with each individual legal jurisdiction regarding the so-called causation threshold definition with regard to causal correlation. For example, in the various different state workers' compensation statutes, there are

D.W. Martin, *Independent Medical Evaluation*,
https://doi.org/10.1007/978-3-319-71906-1_8

some minor differences, and the IME physician is encouraged to understand what the rules are within their individual states that they are dealing with.

Most physicians, when asked to approach a causation question, should apply the traditional causation assessment as established by Austin Bradford Hill. These criteria frequently referred to as the "Bradford Hill Criteria" of causation outline the minimal conditions needed to establish a causal relationship between two occurrences. There are nine criteria that compose the Bradford Hill Criteria. In outlining the Bradford Hill Criteria, it must be understood that it is not about meeting a requisite number of the nine category's criteria that need to be met in order for the threshold of causation to exist, but, rather, it is looked upon in the context of a continuum.

These nine criteria are as follows:

Temporal relationship
Strength of association
Dose-response relationship
Consistency
Plausibility
Consideration of alternate explanations
Experiment
Specificity
Coherence

For more information regarding the Bradford Hill Criteria, we would refer you to the original article that is available free of charge on the Internet at www.edwardtufte.com/tufte/hill.

Thankfully, physicians typically now do not have to look at each individual case and do their own research regarding the various different literature publications that have looked at causal analysis. A landmark textbook published by the American Medical Association entitled the *AMA Guides to the Evaluation of Disease and Injury Causation* now in its second edition, has done a lot of the legwork for physicians in this regard. This textbook takes a rigid approach to qualifying the literature that exists on a variety of different topics. Although the textbook is primarily focused on orthopedic problems, there are chapters that deal with non-musculoskeletal issues. This book can be very helpful and is typically something that each Independent Medical Examining physician should have within their library.

Also, with regard to the causation questions that are asked of Independent Medical Examiners, the subject of apportionment may be critical. Apportionment simply refers to a situation where there may be multiple different reasons for a medical condition to exist. If the IME physician is asked to apportion an injury, what effectively this means is that they are being asked to assign individual percentages of the various different factors that have led to that condition. The problem, of course, is that many medical conditions are multifactorial in their origin. However, even more problematic is the fact that there is virtually no medical literature information that is available to allow the physician to reach an apportionment decision with any degree of surety or clarity. In many cases of an apportioning evaluation, the opinion of the IME physician regarding impairment is relegated to the "educated guess."

Also, it is important for the physician to understand the definition of other terms and phrases that are used in the causation equation. These definitions are:

Exacerbation:
: A temporary worsening of a medical condition which is expected to return to baseline

Aggravation:
: A permanent worsening of an underlying condition which is not going to return to baseline

Acceleration:
: The hastening of the appearance of symptoms of an underlying disease process byan event or exposure

Precipitation:
: The "lighting up" (i.e., an increase in symptoms) of a latent or asymptomatic disease process by an event or exposure

Recurrence:
: The signs or symptoms of a prior illness or injury appearing without a provocative event

Controversial Diagnosis Confirmation

Independent Medical Examiners are oftentimes asked to evaluate individuals who have been given medical diagnoses of which there is a fair debate within the medical community, not only about its existence but, oftentimes, about its appropriate treatment. Such diagnoses include fibromyalgia, complex regional pain syndrome, multiple chemical sensitivities, and chronic fatigue syndrome.

When analyzing these individual conditions, the IME physician should focus specifically on not only the relevant history but also should pay a particular close attention to the concept of the differential diagnosis. Frequently, these controversial diagnoses include criteria that state that the diagnosis can only be given when there is no other medical condition or diagnosis that would better explain the situation. Oftentimes, what the IME physician will find in analyzing these claims is that there is, indeed, a better alternative medical explanation that exists, which may not necessarily have been identified and for which may not necessarily been treated, as opposed to the controversial diagnosis that has been given to the examinee.

The IME physician also should have a very good understanding of the historical explanation regarding these controversial diagnoses.

For example, the American College of Rheumatology, which first published the criteria for fibromyalgia back in the early 1990s, now has promoted a second diagnostic criteria listing for fibromyalgia syndrome that does not even require that a physical examination occur.

Regarding the construct known as complex regional pain syndrome, there have been at least seven different diagnostic criteria that have been published regarding this label since its original inception in 1994. The Center for Disease Control themselves have changed the diagnostic criteria for chronic fatigue syndrome and, as a matter of fact, have also recommended that the nomenclature of the disease be changed. Without keeping up on the historical track record of these various different controversial diagnoses, the IME physician will not have a good basis of knowledge and opinion for which to look at these individual conditions.

Recommendations for Additional Diagnostic Tests and/or Treatment

There is a common question that is posed to the Independent Medical Examiner as to whether or not the examinee requires additional diagnostic testing or whether they require any additional treatment. This, oftentimes, is a corollary to the question about whether the individual has reached a degree of maximum medical improvement.

This type of analysis should be based upon the evidence-based medicine and the literature that has been published with regard to each of the individual conditions.

The IME physician should have ready access to evidence-based treatment guidelines so that they are able to answer this question. It should be noted that just because an examinee has ongoing symptoms and even reports of worsening symptoms, this does not necessarily automatically correlate into the need for additional treatment or for additional testing. There should be an analysis by the IME physician regarding the natural course and progression of the disease process and what a typical expectation is to recovery or not.

Duration of Disability

The Independent Medical Examiner oftentimes is asked about typical durations of individual injuries that might have occurred. For example, in motor vehicle accidents, it is commonly a question as to whether or not the treatment that the examinee has experienced is appropriate. Physicians should have access to databases and evidence-based treatment guidelines that give a reasonable statistical answer to these questions. When answering questions as to whether treatments have been "reasonable and necessary," the physician should not guess but, instead, apply their knowledge and understanding regarding their personal experiences in treating similar conditions and also, then, comparing this to the typical treatment guidelines which are available and published.

Impairment and Maximum Medical Improvement

The IME physician typically is asked to determine impairment ratings, especially within the context of workers' compensation claims. In order for an individual to have an impairment rating, they first must be designated at maximum medical improvement. Maximum medical improvement is that point in time when it is established when no additional medical care is expected to improve the situation. Maximum medical improvement does not mean, however, that maintenance care may not be necessary into the future. Unfortunately, in many claim situations, the designation of maximum medical improvement has been translated into complete claim closure and all care being denied into the future, even that which is reasonable, from the standpoint of ongoing care into the future.

It is not necessarily easy for IME physicians to determine the question regarding maximum medical improvement. In some cases, it is fairly straightforward, such as when one is dealing with a fracture. In other cases, when there is variability to the symptom presentation and impact on activities of daily living that a particular diagnosis may have, it may not necessarily be as straightforward as one would think.

Regarding the issues of impairment rating, the explanation and instruction on how to calculate impairment ratings, based upon the American Medical Association's various books, is beyond the scope of this textbook. If an IME physician needs to become involved in educational activities in order to understand and apply the *AMA Guides to the Evaluation of Permanent Impairment* correctly, then, the physician should be directed to the various different training organizations that are currently in existence that provide these educational experiences. These were previously discussed in Chapter 1.

Level of Disability or Employability

The IME physician is oftentimes asked to comment on the concept of disability. Recall that the definition of "disability" is not the same as the definition of "impairment." Impairment is defined as what is wrong with the individual, whereas disability refers to how the medical condition translates into difficulties with activities of daily living.

Translating the concept of disability into a question of employability also requires due diligence upon the IME physician's part and a reasonably good understanding of the individual work tasks that are being asked about.

There are some individuals who are quite disabled but who are very employable. There are other individuals who have minimal, if any, disability but who might find employability quite a daunting task. Thus, the IME physician should not necessarily make a direct correlation between the two concepts.

When determining whether an examinee is able to return to a particular job task or occupation, the IME physician should perform an analysis using the "risk-capacity-tolerance" paradigm. Physicians are typically very good at determining risk. Usually we are reasonable when it comes to determining capacity. Tolerance is not a scientifically verifiable concept and should not be addressed medically, even though many cases seem to rest within the crosshairs of the determination of tolerance.

Also, the IME physician should be well aware of the medical literature that discusses the long-term health-care outcomes of individuals who are unemployed. There are a variety of medical studies that exist that indicate that work is indeed a positive factor, with regard to an individual's health status. "Worklessness," which is a phrase that is now commonly utilized as opposed to "unemployed," is an individual risk factor for worsening health conditions, including diabetes, heart disease, and cancer. Other negative outcomes associated with worklessness include lower socioeconomic problems, increased divorce rate, poverty, and worsening family dynamics.

Comorbidities

An IME physician is oftentimes asked to pay particular attention to an individual's comorbid medical conditions and how they may affect a specific injury or other illness. This, again, is not an easy task. Some situations are fairly straightforward, such as an individual who has a slow to recover burn injury, who also happens to be an insulin-requiring diabetic. Other conditions are not necessarily as straightforward, such as the implication of heart disease, with regard to the limitation of individuals' exercise capacity and rehabilitation from a spinal injury. The IME physician must utilize their current clinical knowledge in order to answer these questions and also apply whatever evidence-based information that has been published in the medical literature.

Examples

From reviewing several thousand IME reports over 20 plus years, a compilation of usual questions that have been asked by requesting parties has been made. Here are the most common ones.

- Please address the extent of injury.
- Please provide a causal relationship.
- Please determine if treatment is reasonable and/or necessary and related to the on the job injury.
- What future treatment, if any, is reasonable and/or necessary? If so, what type and for what duration of time?
- What medications are reasonable and/or necessary, if any? If so, what type and for what duration?

- Are current medications reasonable and/or necessary? Is there a need for a weaning period?
- What are the long-term side effects of the medications being prescribed/utilized?
- What over-the-counter medications could be utilized?
- Please list typical utilization time frames for any of the prescribed medications/narcotics?
- Based on the objective medical documentation and mechanism of injury, what is the compensable medical diagnosis? Please provide a diagnosis in regard to the work incident.
- Please provide the patient's prognosis in regard to the work-related incident.
- Are current office visits to the treating doctor reasonable and/or necessary?
- Are further testing, diagnostics, durable medical goods, and physical therapy reasonable and/or necessary? If so, please explain.
- Are the diagnostics performed supported by the objective documentation?
- Is the claimant a surgical candidate? If so, is there a need for surgery? What type?
- Is the proposed surgery due to the compensable injury or due to preexisting ordinary disease of life or life processes?
- Is there a need for a second opinion?
- Is there a need for a referral to another physician, specialist, surgeon, etc.?

Bibliography

1. Melhorn M, Talmage J, Ackerman W, Hyman M, editors. AMA guides to the evaluation of disease and injury causation. 2nd ed. Chicago: AMA Press; 2014.
2. Talmage J, Melhorn M, Hyman M, editors. AMA guides to the evaluation of work ability and return to work. 2nd ed. Chicago: AMA Press; 2011.
3. Rondinelli R, editor. AMA guides to the evaluation of permanent impairment. 6th ed. Chicago: AMA Press; 2008.
4. Bradford HA. The environment and disease: association or causation? Proc R Soc Med. 1965;58:295–300. Available from: https://www.edwardtufte.com/tufte/hill.
5. ACOEM Practice Guidelines. 2017. Available from: https://www.mdguidelines.com.
6. Official Disability Guidelines. 2017. Available from: http://www.odg-twc.com.
7. ODG Treatment in Work Comp. 2017. Available from: http://www.odg-twc.com.
8. Wolfe F, Clauw D, Fitzcharles M, Goldenberg D, Häuser W, Katz R, Mease P, Russell A, Russell I, Winfield J. Fibromyalgia criteria and severity scales for clinical and epidemiological studies: a modification of the ACR Preliminary Diagnostic Criteria for Fibromyalgia. J Rheumatol. 2011;38(6):1113–22.
9. Twisk F. A critical analysis of the proposal of the Institute of Medicine to replace myalgic encephalomyelitis and chronic fatigue syndrome by a new diagnostic entity called systemic exertion intolerance disease. Curr Med Res Opin. 2015;31(7):1333–47.
10. Martin D, Barth R, Nguyen T, Randolph D, Talmage J, Travis R. Complex regional pain syndrome – what is the evidence? Chicago: Veritas Medicuss– The AADEP Foundation; 2015.

9 Developing and Authoring an IME Report

This chapter will be devoted to the most important part of the entire IME process, the creation of the report. The IME physician might be a great history taker, might be stellar in the differential diagnostic process, and might even recognized as an expert in their field, but if they unable to write a quality IME report, they will not be seen as helpful. It is often the case that requesting parties have no knowledge about an IME physician other than the quality of the report that they generate.

The simple truth is that physicians typically do not write well. When you think about their formal education process, this might seem a bit difficult to understand, but when you drill down and understand what it entails, it really should not surprise anyone. Physicians by and large tend toward science majors in college, and these bachelor's degree programs at most might require two semesters of English. In medical school, there is virtually no requirement to be able to write well as medical data is now communicated in short factoids. Sometimes, there is a struggle to even find a complete well-written sentence in a student chart note. The problem is that this "habit" typically goes uncorrected. Electronic health records (EHR) do not help this. The plethora of EHRs that are available do not even require the medical student, resident, or practicing physician to write anything in favor of clicking a series of boxes that generate predetermined verbiage. If there is no need for the writing of a sentence let alone a paragraph, laziness sets in. If there is no ability to practice and improve, the writing skill set deteriorates.

But, the stakeholders who are involved in medicolegal claims place a premium upon the written report, where details are pivotal. The ability to clearly communicate a medical history so that anyone reading the report can understand exactly what happened in an injury case becomes not just necessary but critical. Following along the thought processes and understanding how the IME physician has come to their conclusion are held at such a high premium that requesting parties search long and hard to find physicians who possess the ability to write in this manner.

It must be understood that the IME report is a script that may form a foundation for later testimony. Thus, an increased focus upon accuracy and clarity is paramount. Also, IME reports will often become permanent records that will exist in perpetuity. The IME physician should know and prepare for the fact that there is

D.W. Martin, *Independent Medical Evaluation*,
https://doi.org/10.1007/978-3-319-71906-1_9

likely a repository of their saved reports that are being kept in a file somewhere by someone. Legal service companies exist that provide this type of product.

The essential components of a quality IME report can vary but generally should include the following:

Introduction
Results of Clinical Evaluation
Clinical Impressions
Assessment of Current Health Status
Medical Management Plan
Synthesis of Information
Conclusions and Recommendations

Each of these components is best identified within the report by use of subheadings. Given that IME reports are longer than most medical records, the use of subheadings is beneficial as it makes certain sections of information easily identifiable and found. Also, since the report may be read by different people responsible for distinct parts of claim administration, use of subheadings helps those individuals focus on their relevant tasks. For example, the litigator might be interested in the causation section. The nurse case manager might want to look at medical management plan. The insurance company actuary might only be looking at the indemnity costs of disability payments or wage replacement benefits.

Each of these subsections will be reviewed in detail. I am often asked to provide example reports, as it seems that this is most helpful to new physicians performing IMEs, following the medical school educational mantra "see one, do one, teach one." Thus, at the end of this chapter are several examples of reports that I have written. The names in the reports have been changed, but the details have not.

Introduction

The introduction will typically include the identifying information of the examinee which consists of their name, date of birth, and last four digits of their social security number. In some situations, the social security number identifier may not be necessary and in other situations the examinee may not wish to disclose this information, and it is not required to do so. If the claim has been given a case or a file number, it is appropriate to also include this information. In some cases, a date of injury is given to the IME physician; however, I would recommend against using this information in the identifier as there are cases where this date is not really a date of injury but rather the date that a claim has been made or, when in a workers' compensation case, the first report of injury has been filed. Especially in cases where there is a claim of cumulative trauma, the history obtained may show that the onset of symptoms has little correlation with the recorded date of injury. In other situations, the IME physician may find that there is no injury, even if one is claimed.

Within the introductory section, the referral source should be identified to include the specific name of the requesting party as well as the agency or entity that they represent. The purpose of the evaluation should be specifically stated which should include the type of benefit system that the examination is being conducted under as well as any applicable jurisdictional rules that apply. Typically also in the introduction section, there is a reference to the referral letter in so far that it is acknowledged that it has been received and reviewed.

At some point, a listing of all records and radiographs that have been presented for review should be included. It is best to include this list in an appendix that is attached at the end of the IME report as opposed to placing this at the beginning of the report as an extensive list has a tendency to turn off the reader early on if it is done in this manner.

Results of the Clinical Examination

The next portion of the report should include the history and physical examination. When recording the history, some IME physicians prefer to use a sublabel such as "History of Present Illness" or "History of Current Condition." Any such title is appropriate.

Stylistically, the history should tell a story as it is related by the examinee. The narrative of the events should follow the standard approach for all medical histories in that pertinent positives and negatives are to be investigated and recorded.

IME physicians take different approaches regarding how they record the history as it pertains to what is recorded in the past medical records. Some physicians do not include any references to the past records in the history section, preferring to record only the information obtained from the examinee. These reports usually will then include a review of the past records in a different section of the IME report. I have read many of these types of reports, and one of the criticisms against them is that there is a long list of summaries of the medical encounters that can go on for pages and pages. While it is certainly a good idea to review the past records in detail, I find that this approach is unnecessary and actually quite negative in that most requesting parties are well aware of what has occurred previously and do not need to have this degree of detail recounted in an IME report.

Instead of this approach, I favor a different style which incorporates a mixture of what the examinee is reporting to me and what is included in the past medical record. Admittedly, this methodology is more complicated and requires an artistic skill set of writing that is not necessarily easy to master. However, in reviewing this with a host of stakeholders, this method seems to be preferred because it is easier to follow and reads more like a story is being told. This "mixture method" also affords the IME physician the ability to identify not only where the information is coming from (the examinee, the records, or both) but more importantly allows a simplistic method to handle those situations where the history from the examinee does not agree with what is included within the past records. When such disagreement exists, the IME physician should explore this further with the examinee in an attempt to understand the discrepancy. If an explanation is given by the examinee, it should be included here, even if the explanation makes little sense from a medical standpoint.

The history should also include a review of systems plus a listing of current medications and allergies. It is crucial to obtain a detailed occupational history especially when evaluating a disability claim. Family history and social history are just as important. The IME physician should take extra effort to understand the biopsychosocial dynamic of the injury or illness claim. Investigating a history of adverse child events, spousal abuse, or substance abuse can often lead to a better understanding of claim behavior. It also known that one of the strongest predictors of disability claims is the presence of a spouse who is also receiving disability benefits. An understanding of prior workers' compensation claims, including any prior impairment ratings or permanent physical activity restrictions, should be documented in this section. Lastly, a listing of all prior surgeries should be included.

Most IME reports also include a subheading for the physical and/or mental examination results. The IME physical examination must be detailed and thorough, and this should be reflected in the way that it is recorded within the report. Comprehensiveness should rule the process of the examination, and comparison of extremities as well as required range of motion measurements should be noted. If the examination is oriented toward the determination of impairment ratings, a minimum of three trials of range of motion should be recorded as this is a requirement of the *AMA Guides to the Evaluation of Permanent Impairment*. If there are any other unique methods that are required to conduct and record physical examination findings, they should be not only recorded but indicated as such in this section so that there are no questions regarding whether the examination has been conducted under the rules and requirements that the benefit system mandates.

As is the case with any medical evaluation, pertinent positive and negative examination findings specific to the organ system being examined should be listed in detail. For example, there are a number of provocative orthopedic examination maneuvers that are done for several different conditions. Reporting those examination techniques that have been generally accepted as reasonable regarding their sensitivity and specificity of the diagnosis at hand is required. However, this does not mean that the IME physician needs to or should record every examination technique that has ever been published, as many are archaic and have been proven to less appropriate based upon their biostatistical caveats.

A discussion is also relevant here regarding some examination tests that are unique to the specialty or discipline within which they are typically used. The IME physician should be aware of, for example, some of the common chiropractic maneuvers especially if there is a record of them being performed in the prior medical records being reviewed. However, that does not necessarily mean they need to be reproduced because some are not generally recognized as having validity within allopathic or osteopathic practice.

While on the topic of these specific exams, it is recommended that the IME physician incorporate and record the results of what are commonly referred to as validation signs. These signs are usually employed in orthopedic evaluations and are intended to detect the presence of insincere or limited effort. An example of a validation sign are the Waddell's signs, named after Scottish orthopedic surgeon Gordon Waddell, who first published them in 1980 in *Spine*. These signs are intended to detect nonorganic or psychological overlay in individuals with chronic low back pain. Other validation signs include the straight leg raising angle validity test described in the *AMA Guides to the Evaluation of Permanent Impairment, Fifth Edition*, where the tightest supine straight leg angle is compared against the sacral flexion and extension angle when measuring lumbar spinal range of motion.

The seasoned IME physician may employ a set of validation signs that have not yet been formalized within medical textbooks or articles. Some of these examples include the following:

- Comparing examinee supine straight leg test results and symptoms in the context of a dedicated orthopedic exam with a skin or circulation exam of the feet where the examinee unknowingly raises the leg while sitting so the IME physician can have a better look.
- Comparing dedicated shoulder range of motion values recorded with a later neurologic oriented examination of having the examinee hold both arms outstretched or overhead while having their eyes closed to test for palmar or pronator drift.
- Comparing gait patterns when specifically telling the examinee that this is being examined with the gait pattern when the examinee is moving from the chair to the examination table.
- Comparing elbow range of motion values of supination and pronation with the examination of the palm in a seated position for cutaneous or circulation evaluation (Allen's test). A complete palm up position in the seated position with the elbow at a 90° angle equates to 90° of supination of the elbow.

It is also important to record sincerity of effort when testing strength. Items such as breakaway and cogwheeling should be noted. Inconsistencies during the exam with observed events such as opening a door handle to get into or out of the examination room prove useful in determining whether the examinee is portraying a true physiologic or anatomic issue.

It should be known that the physical examination during an IME actually may start before the examinee enters the office. Some IME physicians are fortunate to have their office windows face the parking lot, and observations of gait pattern and methods of getting in and out of a vehicle and how they either are consistent or different with those patterns while in the office are noteworthy. It is relevant to describe how the examinee gets in and out of the chair and off and on the examination table. I have on a few occasions observed claimants who supposedly had severe knee problems kick start their motorcycles with the "injured" leg quite aggressively and normally.

The recording of unusual pain behaviors is necessary as they indicate a situation where there is symptom magnification, inappropriate illness behavior, or possibly even malingering. Items such as inappropriate withdrawal, (some examinees will withdraw an extremity, e.g., before it is even touched by the physician), overt moaning and groaning with simple movements, slow responses to trivial maneuvers, and inappropriate grimacing are examples.

Lastly, regarding the physical examination, the IME physician must know if there are certain methods of performing the examination that are required by the disability system rules. Examples of this might be measuring grip strength using a five-position dynamometer or using Semmes-Weinstein monofilaments to evaluate peripheral nerve sensation.

In this subsection, there should also be a place to discuss the relevant diagnostic tests or radiographs that have been presented as part of the prior records. Most IME physician will discuss these in a separate identifiable part of the report. In some cases, it might be relevant for the IME physician to conduct certain in-office tests. Recall that we previously discussed the potential pitfalls of ordering diagnostic tests as it may be interpreted by some as constituting a physician-patient relationship. However, many IME physicians will perform some simpler tests in their offices especially if the results of those tests are critical in the determination of impairment. Examples of these types of tests done in the office of IME physicians are as follows:

- Pulmonary function tests
- Exercise stress tests
- Spinal X-rays including flexion and extension angles to determine spinal instability
- Visual acuity and visual field testing
- Audiometry
- Certain blood tests if not readily obtainable by other means
- Urine studies

If the IME physician decides to perform these tests, they should understand the technical requirements regarding staff certification necessary to conduct them. Calibration requirements must be strictly followed. The methodology of the testing is typically described in the *AMA Guides to the Evaluation of Permanent Impairment* or within guidelines published by the relevant physician specialty organizations (e.g., American Thoracic Society for PFTs).

Clinical Impressions

The clinical impressions portion of the report is the location where the diagnoses are listed. It is best to list these numerically. This is not the place to use descriptive or causal language as those topics are dealt with in a different section of the report. As an example, a diagnosis should not be listed as "lower back strain leading to chronic pain due to the 2015 motor vehicle accident" but simply "low back strain." Many physicians elect to also include the relevant ICD-10 code, and that is an optional practice.

Assessment of Current Health Status

This section typically includes a section describing prognosis. The IME physician should indicate whether the medical conditions being evaluated are stable, declining, or improving. It is insufficient to simply report this without also going on to explain the medical basis for the opinion. If there are informational items that are missing or diagnostic tests that need to be done to answer this question better, these should be described in detail and the rationale as to why they are necessary.

There are times when the medical condition being evaluated will have a natural and expected deterioration over time. These are most commonly encountered in illness or diagnoses that involve the internal organ systems. This does not preclude the determination and designation of MMI, as we are talking about maximum medical improvement and not maximum medical worsening. The question sometimes comes up as to how these deteriorating medical problems are addressed within disability systems. The answer is that there are usually protocols involved where a claimant can re-file for additional benefits if the condition worsens over time. Thus, it is helpful for the IME physician to comment upon the likelihood of a progressive deterioration of a condition within the report as it helps the requesting party plan for these contingencies in the future.

It is important for the IME physician to understand that there are now several scientific studies that have addressed health status in individuals who are not working. Such "worklessness" has been shown to worsen (or even increase the incidence of) several chronic medical conditions including diabetes, cancer, coronary artery disease, and a variety of mental health conditions. When assessing an individual who has been out of work or one who might not be working into the future, it is relevant to include this vital information.

Medical Management Plan

This section deals with the recommendations for future further evaluations and a treatment plan. In cases where an examinee is at maximum medical improvement, a statement regarding whether there is no additional care recommended as opposed to a need for ongoing maintenance care should be explained. It is extremely helpful to the requesting party for the IME physician to describe maintenance care recommendations in detail, listing the frequency of need for physician or other ancillary health-care provider visits, the duration of medication need, and the requirements of replacement of prosthetic or medical care devices (ambulatory assistive devices, braces, etc.).

It is also helpful to discuss the time frames that will be required to accomplish the treatments that are being recommended. If a surgery is being suggested, normal postsurgical healing periods should be included along with any expected postsurgical care processes. Surgical complications should be discussed if they are unique or pertinent to the decision process or if the surgery is controversial or optional. Also, it is helpful to include expectations of future health-care needs if a surgery is declined or does not occur for a different reason.

If certain therapies are being suggested, the number of treatments and time frames over which they should occur should be included. If a mental health issue is being addressed, it may be appropriate to discuss the differences between options for care between psychiatrists, psychologists, or other mental health providers.

The reason why it is important to include this level of detail is that the requesting party is often in need of making appropriate set-aside determinations or plans for future incurred medical expenses. Obviously there can be great differences in cost when comparing a surgical case versus one that can be managed with conservative care.

Synthesis of Information

This section of the report often will include the "meat" or "crux" of the issues that the IME physician is being asked to address. Depending upon what the focus of the IME is, there may be extended discussions regarding causation, impairment, disability, or return to work recommendations. With comprehensive IMEs, each of these might be included, and it is suggested that they each be given their own section and subheading.

In the following chapter, we will address these individual topics in more detail. It is within this section that it is common to list reference material that supports your opinion. Some IME reports use footnotes, but I believe that it is a better strategy to list the reference work within the body of the report as it has a tendency to give your opinion more force.

There are times when the IME physician may not have enough medical information in order to answer a question that is posed. The evaluator must be honest when this occurs and not rush to judgment. If there are additional tests that are needed, they should be explained as to what they will help determine. If a different specialty evaluation is needed, the specific issues that the specialist should address should be described.

Within this section, the IME physician must review and analyze all of the available documentation and ask whether it fits with the examinee's story or not. Many times, there will be inconsistencies, and the evaluator should not only describe these but attempt to determine the reasons why.

Frequently, the IME physician will be asked about the appropriateness of treatment that has occurred to date. Such questions are usually framed as whether the treatment has been "reasonable and necessary." It is here that evidence-based treatment guidelines can be referenced as they provide the backdrop for answering these questions.

In cases of long-term disability determination, the IME physician should expressly state if the examinee meets the requirements of disability that is stated within the policy. Of course, this requires that the examiner have a good knowledge of what those requirements are. Since there can be variability between disability systems, a detailed working understanding is paramount.

Conclusion and Recommendations

The final section of the IME report includes concluding remarks and specific answers to the questions that have been posed by the requesting party. It is recommended that the IME report repeat and list the questions verbatim and that clear and complete answers be given.

It is critical that all the IME physician's opinions be given "within a reasonable degree of medical certainty," which is the legal standard that must be met for those opinions to be considered and entered as part of legal testimony.

Lastly, the IME physician is wise to include disclaimers at the end of the report. These disclaimers allow the IME physician latitude in changing their opinion if additional medical records are found that were not previously presented or if new medical facts are obtained. They also re-enforce the fact that there is not a doctor-patient relationship and that the opinions given in the report are not intended to necessarily be acted upon because the IME physician is not the treating doctor. The disclaimers also point out that the IME physician opinions are not intended to substitute for a legal opinion or for an administrative act to be made or enforced. These last points are critical to avoid the situation where an IME physician is accused of being "judge and jury" regarding the claim that is being evaluated.

Included in the appendix to this chapter are examples of IME disclaimers that can be used within reports. Originally developed by Gary Freeman MD JD, a long-standing faculty member within AADEP, they can be adjusted to serve the needs of the individual IME physician within their jurisdiction. They have proved to be invaluable in certain cases where the IME physician has been taken to task by attorneys who attempt to show that the opinions of the IME physician have been used to harm their clients.

Today, it is usually not difficult to find the IME physician that has been selected by the requesting party. However, some IME physicians travel to provide their services in different areas, so it is always a good idea to include within the report the methodology to contact the IME physician if there are additional questions or inquiries that the requesting party wishes to make.

The IME report should always be signed by the IME physician after proper proofreading and correction. It is not acceptable to send a report without a signature or to use a stamp that states "sent unreviewed (or unsigned) to avoid delay." Such practices do not project professionalism and credibility and are to be avoided.

Stylistic Issues and Artistic Points

This text cannot teach the budding IME physician English, grammar, or basics of composition. Having said that, it is my impression that a substantial number of physicians simply do not write well. Since that is the case, there are several helpful hints and artistic recommendations that are worthwhile pointing out.

The written report projects your credibility. Requesting parties may know nothing about you other than what they receive in the mail. Whether that sounds crass or not is irrelevant, because the report that you submit will definitely be read by many individuals. As such, it is the best advertisement that you can accomplish if you are trying to build your IME practice. The report's quality is the single most important driver in marketing your performance as an IME physician.

Do not think for a minute that IME physicians operate in a bubble. Claims adjusters, nurse case managers, attorneys, and other stakeholders that utilize IMEs talk among themselves. They do it informally as well as formally. If you do a good job with your IME reports, I can guarantee you that you will receive requests from other parties. Word-of-mouth advertising will take care of itself.

So what makes a good IME report read well? It should be written in a style that will stimulate the reader. Many claims examiners or attorneys may be reading your report as the tenth one during that day. The idea is that the IME reports should tell a story and move the reader forward. As you read the report, you should get the sensation and the feeling that you want to get to the next section eagerly.

But, when writing IME reports, the physician should understand the level of expertise of the reader. Writing at a level that only physicians would be able to understand would be pointless. Although it is acceptable to include proper medical terminology in the physical exam and diagnostic section, the history and discussion sections should generally be written using lay terminology that most in the public would be able to understand. If medical terms must be used, consider defining them in a glossary.

It is often asked what tone the report should have. This is an excellent question, and there are different opinions on the question because it depends upon how the report is going to be used. Some IME requestors might want a report that has a certain degree of "shock value" if it is going to be used to argue for or against a contentious topic. Nevertheless, in general it is best to write in a relaxed tone. If there is a feeling when reading the report that someone is shouting at you, chances are the verbiage is too aggressive.

In addition to the traditional teaching points of paying attention to sentence and paragraph length, verb tense consistency is critical. One way of determining whether your report is easy to read is to read it out loud yourself. If something does not sound right, it needs to be revised.

Analogies usually are not useful in IME reports as the specificity of the medical issues typically preclude their utility. However, there may be a role for them in the discussion section if the IME physician feels that it could drive a point home.

As has been previously discussed in earlier chapters, these examinations do not establish a physician-patient relationship. The report should never use the term "patient" as there could be a question that this relationship has been established when other measures have been taken to preclude it. Additionally, other sections of the report should avoid discussions of treatment that are in the active voice. For example, in discussing a potential treatment for a peripheral neuropathy, the writer should not say "This examinee should be treated by starting oral gabapentin," but rather "One of the considerations in additional treatment for peripheral neuropathy is gabapentin" thus avoiding any possible inference of treatment from the IME physician.

The report should avoid redundancies. IME doctors seem to have a lot of trouble with this. State your point once and then move on. Junk words or use of the "phrase of the day" is unnecessary. The use of clichés or "doctorisms" which are phrases commonly used among our profession that the lay public does not understand should obviously not be used. An example of this that I once read where the IME physician was trying to make a point that there were too many diagnostic tests being done, stated, "the treating physician might as well order a porcelain titer." While that might bring a chuckle to doctors, the lay public might think that something like that actually exists.

One area that I would guard against is the tendency to fall into the use of template or boilerplate reports. While it is fine for the IME physician to use a standard approach for report creation and subheadings, using similar sentences or language across different reports should be avoided. When requesting parties look at several IME reports from the same physician, if they all look the same, read the same and contain the same sentences, it will look like the IME physician is doing nothing more than churning out written work without bothering to think about what is being communicated.

IME physicians are sometimes asked to comment on financial estimates of care. I believe that this should be avoided. For one thing, doctors usually are not trained in medical pricing or economics. Additionally, there may be too wide a range of health-related costs for a given examinee condition to really make sense out of it. When asked this question, it is best to suggest that a billing or health-care cost expert be consulted, unless, of course, the IME physician has some specific training in that area that would otherwise allow them to answer.

The last area that I will address is the use of what I call "no-no words." I call them this because they are either unnecessary or inflammatory and do not add anything to a sentence. But, I find they appear in IME reports quite often. Here is this list.

- Whatsoever
- Totally
- Absolutely
- Whatever
- Like
- Completely
- Blatant
- Basically
- Essentially
- Clearly
- Entirely
- Very

Examples and Exercises

The practical experience of writing your first IME report can be a scary proposition. Over and over I am asked to provide example reports so that the beginning physician has at least something to refer to. At the end of this chapter, there are several examples of IME reports. All of the identifying information within those reports are fictional.

I have also included an exercise on how an average report can be turned into an excellent report. As part of the educational process of teaching physicians about IMEs, prior courses have included writing exercises that work on the finer points of report generation. This is also included so that you can see how some of the stylistic issues that have been discussed in this chapter can be applied.

The final item that is included at the end of this chapter is the former gradation scheme used by the American Academy of Disability Evaluating Physicians when peer reviewing IME reports that were required for attaining the degree of fellow. While no longer used by AADEP (now IAIME) for fellowship determination, several IME physicians have found this to be a useful reference when self-critiquing their own reports.

Appendix 1: Three Sample Disclaimers

These are three sample disclaimers which I find useful for incorporation in the medical report

- The opinions rendered in this case are the opinions of this evaluator. This evaluation has been conducted on the basis of the medical examination and documentation as provided, with the assumption that the material is true and correct. If more information becomes available at a later date, an additional service/report/reconsideration may be requested. Such information may or may not change the opinions rendered in this evaluation. This opinion is based on a clinical assessment, examination, and documentation. This opinion does not constitute per se a recommendation for specific claims or administrative functions to be made or enforced.
- This Independent Medical Evaluation is based upon the subjective complaints, history given by the patient, the objective medical records and tests provided to me, and the physical findings of the patient. Impairment ratings are given according to the Guides to the Evaluation of Permanent Impairment, Fourth Edition, American Medical Association. Recommendations regarding work and impairment ratings are given totally independently of the requesting agents. The opinions are based upon reasonable medical probability. Medicine is both an art and a science and although a patient may appear to be fit for return to duty there is no guarantee that the patient will not be reinjured or suffer additional injury once he returns. If further information is required please contact the undersigned.
- The opinions rendered in this case are the opinions of the reviewer. The review has been conducted without a medical examination of the individual reviewed. The review is based on documents provided with the assumption that the material is true and correct. If more information becomes available at a later date, an additional service/report/reconsideration may be requested. Such information may or may not change the opinions rendered in this report. This report is a clinical assessment of documentation and the opinions are based on the information available. This opinion does not constitute per se a recommendation for specific claims or administrative functions to be made or enforced.

Freeman G. Tips for writing reports. Conference proceedings of the AADEP Comprehensive Training Course. 31 March 1998. Chicago. Chicago: American Academy of Disability Evaluating Physicians

Appendix 2: Example IME Reports

January 8, 2008

RITA SMITH, RN
MEDICAL CASE MANAGEMENT NURSE
BASS & HALIBUT COMPANIES
P.O. BOX 2201
OCEAN CITY, IA 51104

RE: Processor Watson
SS#: xxx-xx-9170
DOB: 12/18/1982

Dear Ms. Smith:

Please be advised that I had the opportunity to evaluate the above named individual at my office at 4230 War Eagle Drive in Sioux City, Iowa for purposes of an Independent Medical Examination on January 8, 2008.

Please be advised the examinee read, understood and signed the notice of informed consent for Independent Medical Evaluation and this was placed in her chart.

Please also be advised that I had an opportunity to review pertinent past medical records surrounding her claim of injury to her low back. The following constitutes a medical record source list:

1. Medical records from Richard J. Klein, D.O. of the St. Luke's Center for Occupational Health Excellence
2. Medical records from Leonel Hightower, M.D., neurologist affiliated with the Tri-State Orthopedic group
3. Medical records from Steven J. Shocker, M.D. of the Center for Awesomeness.
4. Physical therapy records from Physical Therapy Guys, P.C.
5. Physical therapy records from Sioux City Physical Therapy
6. Physical therapy records from the Center for Neurosciences, Orthopaedics and Spine, P.C.
7. Medical records from Eric Heiden, D.O., Radiology Department, St. Luke's Regional Medical Center
8. Functional Capacity Examination Report from Marcus Witbier of Witbier Workforce Assessment, L.L.C.
9. Procedure note from Paul Burke, D.O., from the Pierce Street Same Day Surgery Center, L.C.

There are additional records surrounding her care which are not available, but are known to exist, which include those from the following source:

1. Chiropractic records from Fluent Chiropractic Center

PROCESSOR WATSON
1/08/08
PAGE 2

History of Present Illness

Ms. Processor Watson is a 25-year-old white female who presents herself today at the request of Rita J. Smith, RN, nurse case management nurse affiliated with Bass & Halibut, at the behest of CCMSI Insurance Company, for purposes of an Independent Medical Evaluation surrounding complaints of back pain stemming from a work related incident that occurred on February 1, 2007.

She explains that she was working for Sunrise Retirement Center and was helping to lift a resident from a wheelchair to a bed, with the assistance of another Certified Nursing Assistant. Both coworkers attempted to lift the resident underneath each opposing arm, but when Ms. Watson attempted to do this, she strained her back experiencing not pain right away, but approximately 5 to 10 minutes after the incident. She described the initial pain as sharp and stabbing, and on the left side of the low back.

She presented to Dr. Richard Klein of the St. Luke's Center for Occupational Health Excellence for treatment on February 8, 2007 initially with a diagnosis of lumbar strain. She was treated with conservative measures, including Tylenol, Flexeril and physical therapy. She was placed on restricted duty.

The lady was followed up on February 19, 2007 and, again on March 5, 2007 and March 19, 2007 with continuation of conservative based care and the same medications.

When she returned for a follow up visit on April 2, 2007, she was referred to Neurology for further evaluation and treatment, as she continued to have complaints of lower back discomfort.

She was seen by Dr. Leonel Hightower, who suggested MRI scanning, as well as an epidural corticosteroid injection and other medications, including Amitriptyline, Mobic and Ultram. The MRI scan showed degenerative disk changes at the L5-S1 level, but no impact upon the exiting nerve roots or impact upon the spinal cord.

It is a little bit unclear as to the events, with respect to her injections, in that the documentation indicates a June 8, 2007 leftward sacroiliac joint injection performed by Dr. Luebbert, as opposed to an epidural injection. Ms. Watson indicates that she received approximately 1 week's worth of improvement of her symptoms after that injection, only to have this return to baseline.

Dr. Hightower did not have any other recommendations, other than continuing with conservative based measures. The lady was then, apparently, evaluated by Dr. Fluent of Fluent Chiropractic and had a treatment attempt at chiropractic measures. I do not have any chiropractic notes to know specifically the content or the duration of the chiropractic intervention, but apparently this did not alleviate any of her symptoms either.

She was eventually forwarded by Dr. Fluent on to Dr. Steven Shocker, who saw her and also felt that she did not have a surgical lesion. He suggested continued conservative measures.

PROCESSOR WATSON
1/08/08
PAGE 3

She had an epidural corticosteroid injection performed by Dr. Paul Burke in November of 2007. She indicates that gave no relief whatsoever, even for a short duration of time.

It is my understanding that Dr. Shocker did not have any other recommendations for treatment. Dr. Klein also got back into the evaluation process in late November and early December of 2007 suggesting a Functional Capacity Examination and Independent Medical Examination.

A Functional Capacity Examination performed by Marcus Witbier of Witbier Workforce Assessment dated December 13, 2007 indicates an invalid Functional Capacity Examination with passage of only 39 percent of the validity criteria.

In speaking with Ms. Watson today, she continues to complain of low back pain, left side of mid line and the lower portion of her lumbar spine. She denies any current radiation of pain into the legs, nor does she complain of any numbness or tingling into the legs.

She does not complain of any type of bowel or bladder function abnormalities.

She notes that she occasionally will have difficulties with her sleep quality, but not consistently so.

As far as her work activities are concerned, she has been on a transitional duty situation where she basically is only doing portions of her job, including dining activities.

Review of Systems

Her Review of Systems is positive for having a history of hospitalization for pyelonephritis in December of 2006 and January of 2007.

The remainder of the Review of Systems is negative except for that described above.

Past Medical History

Current Medications: Include Mobic 7.5 mg. q. day; Tramadol 50 mg. q. 4 to 6 hours p.r.n; Extra Strength Tylenol, 1 q. 4 to 6 hours p.r.n; Amitriptyline 10 mg., 2 tablets q. h.s.

Allergies: To sulfa and morphine sulfate

Family History	: Positive for hypertension.
Social History	: Reveals that this lady smokes approximately 1/2-pack of cigarettes daily. She denies alcohol or illicit drug use.
Occupational History	: Reveals that she has worked as a Certified Nursing Assistant for 6 years. She has been at Sunrise Retirement Center for 5 years and prior to that, at Indian Hills Nursing and Rehab Center for 1-1/2 years.
Surgical History	: Positive for a laparoscopic appendectomy.

PROCESSOR WATSON
1/08/08
PAGE 4

Radiographs Available for My Review

I have no radiographs that have been made available for my review, other than the plain film x-rays that were taken by Dr. Klein. I find no specific or concerning abnormalities on those films.

She, apparently, has had a bone scan in addition to the lumbosacral spine MRI scan. I only have those Radiology reports. The Radiology reports would suggest that the MRI scan showed degenerative disk desiccation at L5-S1 with degenerative protrusions with no evidence of herniation or impact upon the exiting nerve roots or spinal cord. There, apparently, was some question on the bone scan of a vertebral body abnormality, but this is relatively unremarkable and not correlated on the MRI scan imaging.

Physical Examination

The lady was pleasant and cooperative during the course of the history taking and physical examination. She was able to get on and off the examination table in no acute distress.

In the seated position, her straight leg and crossed straight leg raise tests were negative.

Her lower extremity strength revealed 5/5 strength using manual muscle testing protocols of the dorsiflexors and plantar flexors of the feet, as well as the quadriceps and the hamstrings.

There was no muscular tone loss, atrophic change or spasm of the lower extremity musculature.

Calf circumferences measured 10 centimeters below the tibial tubercle were equal bilaterally at 36 centimeters.

Light touch and two-point discrimination testing of the lower extremities were well within normal limits.

There is no evidence of any clubbing, cyanosis or edema. Peripheral pulses were normal.

Lumbosacral spine inclinometry was performed. The following measured values were obtained:

Lumbar flexion	45 degrees
Lumbar extension	20 degrees
Right lateral flexion	20 degrees
Left lateral flexion	25 degrees

Her supine straight leg raise test on the left was 70 degrees and on the right was 75 degrees.

PROCESSOR WATSON
1/08/08
PAGE 5

Waddell's testing was performed which revealed no representation of pain with simulated rotation or axial compression. There were no nonanatomic descriptors of pain. There was no hypersensitivity noted. There were no significant differences between supine versus seated straight leg raise tests.

Palpably, she did complain of tenderness upon palpation over the left parasacral area. There is no sacroiliac joint or sciatic notch tenderness appreciated. The Faber's testing was negative.

Her gait pattern reveals retained capabilities with heel-toe and tandem gait. There is no antalgic posturing noted.

Assessment

(1) Mechanical low back pain

Prognosis

This lady's prognosis is **good**.

Recommendations

The evidence based medical recommendations, at this point, for this lady's complaints of back pain would be to continue with a home based exercise program concentrating on flexibility, strengthening and aerobic-type of activity.

Concerning medication treatment, the evidence based medical protocols and literature would strongly suggest management of her back pain, at this point, with over-the-counter analgesic medications, either in the form of Acetaminophen or Ibuprofen, or a combination of those two. Long term utilization of muscle relaxant medications and pain medications are not supported by the literature.

She does not need any further diagnostic testing.

She is not a surgical candidate.

There is no indication, at this point, for additional injection therapy, such as epidural corticosteroid injection, sacroiliac joint injection, or facet injection.

The evidence based medical literature would strongly support resumption of normal activity.

Causation

Causation, in this case, is based upon the medical evidence as presented in the record, as well as interview with the examinee. Her current back pain situation does have direct causal correlation to the work related lifting incident that occurred on February 1, 2007.

PROCESSOR WATSON
1/08/08
PAGE 6

Impairment

Impairment rating, in this case, is based upon the principles of the AMA Guides to the Evaluation of Permanent Impairment, Sixth Edition.

This lady's impairment rating would be based upon the Spinal Chapter, which is Chapter 17 of the AMA Guides, Sixth Edition.

Concerning the lumbar spine, one would specifically review the spine regional grid system, which is contained within Table 17-4 on page 570. This lady would meet the Class 1 descriptor under Nonspecific Chronic or Chronic Recurrent Low Back Pain. The default value for the CDX designation within this Class is 2 percent.

The adjustment score for the functional history is taken from Table 17-6 and is consistent with a Grade 3 modifier of pain and symptoms with less than normal activity. Her Grade modifier for physical examination, taken from Table 17-7 on page 576 is a Grade 0. Her Grade Modifier for Clinical Studies, taken from Table 17-9 on page 581 is somewhat difficult to interpret. There is no possibility for the physician to use a Grade Modifier 1; however, when presented with this dilemma, one needs to pick a side, so to speak, with respect to either utilization of Grade 0 or Grade 2. I am arguing for utilizing Grade 2 modifier because of the MRI findings of the L5-S1 degenerative condition not being clinically insignificant and certainly not being consistent with this individual's age. Therefore, I think a Grade 2 modifier is appropriate.

In calculating the Net Adjustment Score utilizing the instructions on page 582, this would yield a -1 Net Adjustment, which would place this lady within a Grade B designation of Class 1.

Turning back to Table 17-4 on page 570, this would, therefore, yield a 1 percent whole person permanent partial impairment rating.

This lady has reached a degree of maximum medical improvement.

Return to Work Issues

The current evidence based medical literature on this lady's clinical condition strongly suggests return to normal activities.

We have a Functional Capacity Examination which has been performed, which is invalid. The examinee was willing to show us only a sedentary light physical demand level and the physical therapist administering this test felt that she should be able to work at least at a light medium physical demand level with the recommendation that her true functional capabilities must be left to professional conjecture.

PROCESSOR WATSON
1/08/08
PAGE 7

I would indicate that professional conjecture, although typically somewhat argumentative and difficult to understand previously, has now become more clear-cut with advanced scientific studies on chronic low back pain, which clearly show that an individual does better with long term outcomes if they are told to resume normal activities. Therefore, I do not believe that this lady should be placed on any permanent physical restrictions and should be encouraged to return to her normal activities.

Conclusion

The above statements have been made with a reasonable degree of medical certainty/probability.

The opinions rendered in this case are the opinion of this evaluator. This evaluation has been conducted on the basis of medical examination and documentation as provided, with the expectation this material is true and correct. If more information becomes available at a later date, an additional service/report/reconsideration may be requested. Such information may or may not change the opinions rendered in this evaluation. This opinion is based on clinical assessment, examination and documentation. This opinion does not constitute, per se, recommendations for specific claims or administrative functions to be made or enforced.

If you have any questions with respect to this evaluation, please contact me personally through the office.

Sincerely,

Douglas W. Martin, MD, FACOEM, FAADEP, FAAFP, CIME, CEDIR

Fellow, American College of Occupational & Environmental Medicine
Fellow, American Academy of Disability Evaluating Physicians
Fellow, American Academy of Family Physicians
Certified Independent Medical Examiner (ABIME)
Certified Evaluator of Disability & Impairment Rating (AADEP)

DWM/lap

March 21, 2011

CHRIS J. ATTORNEY
ATTORNEY WORLD P.C.
225 SECOND STREET, SE, SUITE 200
P.O. BOX 36
CEDAR CREEK, NE 68037

RE: Valorie Grant
SS#: XXX-XX-1052
DOB: 11/07/1953

Dear Mr. Attorney:

Please be advised that I had the opportunity to evaluate the above named individual at my office at 4230 War Eagle Drive in Sioux City, Iowa for purposes of an Independent Medical Examination on March 21, 2011.

Please be advised that the examinee read, understood and signed the notice of informed consent for Independent Medical Evaluation and this was placed in her chart.

Thank you for your letter dated March 16, 2011 that summarizes this lady's claim history and includes questions that you need to have addressed. Accompanying this letter are pertinent past medical records and other information sources what I have reviewed in preparation of this report. Please see Appendix A for a listing of these pieces of correspondence.

History of Present Illness

Ms. Valorie Grant is a 57-year-old white female who presents herself today for an Independent Medical Examination, at the request of Chris J. Attorney, attorney-at-law, surrounding claims of injury to her right shoulder. The letter that I have received from Mr. Attorney would also seem to imply that she is claiming a back injury. However, when I reviewed this with the claimant today, she seemed extremely surprised about any spinal problems and stated that it was her understanding that the issue was simply with respect to her right shoulder.

This lady reports that she believes that she began to experience problems with respect to right shoulder pain several years ago (she is unable to give me a specific date) where she was carrying a tray of food into a freezer at her work place, known as Timmy's Catering, when she had a slip injury and fell with her right arm into a rack. She, apparently, did not go all the way to the ground. The medical record would suggest that this incident was taken care of by Dr. Strittholt in 2005, wherein his record would indicate an evaluation on October 24, 2005, which resulted in treatment with a shoulder injection.

The lady reports that she did have good improvement with respect to the injection, at that point. The medical record would also suggest that the lady underwent advanced diagnostic imaging of her right shoulder with an MRI scan on November 15, 2005 showing mild acromioclavicular joint hypertrophy and degenerative changes with tendinosis.

VALORIE GRANT
3/21/11
PAGE 2

Over the course of the next several years, the lady then states that she had on and off exacerbations of right shoulder pain. The medical record would suggest that yearly thereafter she presented back to Dr Strittholt for right shoulder pain which was basically treated with repeat injections. This was done in 2006 and then also again in 2007. In early 2008, she had another reported problem of exacerbation which was treated with injection and then the lady had another problem of reexacerbation in October of 2008 which led to yet another injection. However, apparently, that did not necessarily improve her symptoms, as it had prior. In April of 2009 she had more problems and a repeat MRI scan was done. Partial thickness tearing of the rotator cuff appeared to be present with, again, the acromioclavicular joint hypertrophy, which was noted on the prior MRI scan. An extensive tendinitis signal was noted.

After this point in time, there was some discussion about options for care. But, eventually, on July 21, 2009, the lady underwent a shoulder arthroscopic procedure. A subacromial decompression with rotator cuff repair was performed.

The lady, apparently, did reasonably well with surgery, but in discussion with her today, she reports that it took longer than what she had hoped. She states that she had some postoperative physical therapy that was helpful.

She reports that she continues to have some degree of issues concerning her right shoulder. She reports that it is better with the surgery than what it was. The main issue that she seems to have is with respect to overhead type of activity with her right arm. She states that she is unable to lift as much as she used to be able to lift with her right arm. She reports difficulty with household chores, such as vacuuming. She has had significant improvement in problems with nighttime wakening, and that is not really a substantial issue for her presently. She does state that she awakens sometimes with stiffness in the right shoulder.

She denies any substantial numbness or tingling that follows a dermatomal distribution. She does not report any crepitus into the shoulder joint currently. She denies any type of headache symptomatology.

Upon questioning, she specifically denies any current neck, thoracic or lumbar pain.

Review of Systems

This lady's Review of Systems reveals that she has no reported active medical problems.

Past Medical History

Current Medications: Include a calcium supplement, a multivitamin and Effexor (unknown dose q. day).

VALORIE GRANT
3/21/11
PAGE 3

Allergies: None

Family History	: Positive for cancer and diabetes mellitus.
Occupational History	: Reveals that this lady worked for Timmy's Catering for a period of 20 years with the last date of employment being July 21, 2009. She began working for Floyd Valley Hospital as a cook in December of 2009, where she continues to work today.
Social History	: Reveals that this lady smokes 2-packs of cigarettes weekly. She denies alcohol or illicit drug use.
Surgical History	: Positive for 2 C-Sections and a cystoscopy.
Prior Medical Intervention	: The medical record presented suggests that this lady has had back and neck problems that have been evaluated by chiropractic. She has also had prior low back pain evaluated by primary care physicians at Medical Associates in 2002. There is a listing in September of 2003 from Krull Chiropractic of pain in the trapezius and the posterior right shoulder.

Radiographs Available for My Review

None.

Physical Examination

The lady was pleasant and cooperative during the course of the history taking and physical examination. She was able to get in and out of the chair, off and on the examination table, and move about the room with no difficulty.

Examination of her right shoulder reveals that there is a 7 centimeter scar which is located in somewhat of a curvilinear, horizontal location in the anterior aspect of her upper right arm. I am assuming that this is from the previous surgical intervention.

Palpably, she complains of no tenderness over the collar bone, over the acromioclavicular joint, over the biceps tendon, or of the subacromial bursa. She has mild tenderness upon palpation over the medial superior scapular border at the insertion of the levator scapular muscle. There is no scapular winging, however. There is no tenderness over the rhomboid, nor over the trapezius or the cervical structures.

The reflexes of the biceps, brachioradialis and triceps are 2+ and symmetric. Light touch and two-point discrimination testing are well within normal limits.

Confrontation strength testing reveals 5/5 strength concerning dorsal interosseous, grip strength and wrist deviator strength bilaterally. There is, likewise, 5/5 strength concerning bilateral biceps and triceps strength.

VALORIE GRANT
3/21/11
PAGE 4

There is 5/5 strength bilaterally in the shoulder with flexion, extension, internal and external rotation and adduction. The right shoulder does show, however, 4+/5 strength with lateral abduction, whereas, on the left, this is 5/5.

There is no evidence of any muscle tone loss, atrophic change or spasm of the upper extremity musculature. There is no muscle tone loss, atrophic change or spasm of the posterior shoulder girdle or over the paracervical musculature.

Range of motion examination of the shoulders was then performed utilizing the goniometric protocols described in the Fifth Edition of the AMA Guides to the Evaluation of Permanent Impairment. The range of motion values are as follows:

Right

Flexion	130 degrees
Extension	50 degrees
Internal rotation	60 degrees
External rotation	75 degrees
Abduction	120 degrees
Adduction	60 degrees

Left

Flexion	140 degrees
Extension	75 degrees
Internal rotation	70 degrees
External rotation	90 degrees
Abduction	140 degrees
Adduction	60 degrees

No other abnormalities are noted.

Assessment

1. History of right shoulder impingement syndrome
2. Status post multiple injections and eventually decompression operation for #1 above.

Prognosis

This lady's prognosis is **good**.

Recommendations

I have no additional medical care recommendations for Ms. Grant.

I do not believe that she requires additional diagnostic testing, medication prescriptions, injections or surgical intervention concerning her right shoulder.

VALORIE GRANT
3/21/11
PAGE 5

Causation

Causation, in this case, is based upon a review of the medical documentation as presented, as well as interview with the examinee.

This has been applied to current evidence based medicine in the form of medical literature published concerning the issue of causation analysis for shoulder impingement problems.

It is recognized by this examiner that there is some degree of differences of opinion within Dr. Strittholt's notes of whether or not he either feels or does not feel that her right shoulder issues have some contribution of work relatedness. Early on, it appears as though his opinion is more on the line that this was a degenerative process; but then, towards the end of the treatment protocol, he seems to change his opinion a bit, thinking that this is either an aggravation or exacerbation. I admit that it is somewhat difficult to follow his thought processes as they change throughout the years.

It is also recognized that Dr. Brian Johnson, who is an Orthopedic Surgeon affiliated with the Center for Neurosciences, Orthopedics and Spine, P.C. was apparently asked to do an Independent File Review by a claims manager concerning this, and has given the opinion that he feels it is not work related and only a degenerative process.

I do not have a formal job description that has been presented to me for this lady's work activities at Timmy's Catering. Given her description to me today of what this company does, which is primarily provide catering for a variety of different social functions in the LeMars and surrounding area, including things such as graduations, weddings, class reunions, business trips, etc., she reports that primarily her job was food preparation and transport. From her deposition transcript, it appears that the main issues that she was having at the work place was pain concerning stirring of pots and also chopping vegetables and fruits.

Applying the evidence based medicine causation analysis, as well as the principles of the Bradford-Hill causation analysis protocol indicates that the medical literature suggests that individuals have to have a combination of risk factors for rotator cuff tendinitis or impingement syndrome to have a relationship to work activities. The combination of risk factors can be repetitive, from the standpoint of overhead activities, as well as with awkward postures, or with respect to vibratory insult with overhead reaching, etc.

Concerning the issue of upper arm positioning, the medical literature would suggest that individuals need to have repetitive lateral abduction-type of postures greater than 70 degrees in order for work to be assigned a causal contribution.

Given my knowledge of what this lady is describing to me, with respect to her catering job, and also based upon her deposition transcript, as well as upon a review of the medical documentation, it is my opinion that her work activities are insufficient to be able to assign a contribution cause to the issue of shoulder impingement.

As is more typically true than not, individuals who have shoulder impingement follow a continuum of problems over years. With respect to her diagnostic imaging,

VALORIE GRANT
3/21/11
PAGE 6

which shows acromioclavicular joint hypertrophy with a small inferior spur and the original MRI scan of 2005, which shows not much space in the subacromial bursa, typically, the tendon first is impinged by the bony structures and then subsequently, just as a rope has a nick put on it and continues to fray over time, it becomes thin to the point where a partial tear develops and then, in some individuals, a full thickness tear. This continuum, however, is a natural part of the aging process and only in a situation where there is a clear or traumatic event or substantial combination of risk factors, as is described above, can a work causation contribution be assigned to the problem.

I, therefore, have a tendency to agree with Dr. Johnson's Independent File Review concerning the causation analysis.

Furthermore, I would note that, on physical examination today, this lady does have some limitation of range of motion and does not have "normal" range of motion concerning the unaffected left shoulder. This is further evidence that the degenerative process has a more stronger association with these types of issues.

Impairment

Impairment rating, in this case, is based upon the principles of the AMA Guides to the Evaluation of Permanent Impairment, Fifth Edition, as well as the principles and practices and utilization of those Guides, as taught by the American Academy of Disability Evaluating Physicians and as tested by that organization, as well as that by the American Board of Independent Medical Examiners.

It is unclear to me the basis for the previous impairment rating of Dr. Strittholt, which apparently is 12 percent of the upper extremity.

Proper application of the AMA Guides, Fifth Edition is to calculate this lady's impairment rating based upon the range of motion figures, which appear on page 476, 477 and 479, respectively.

It is incorrect to assign any additional impairment above and beyond this for any type of strength loss, as the AMA Guides, Fifth Edition strength section clearly indicates, on page 508, that decreased strength can not be rated in the presence of decreased motion, painful conditions, deformities, or absence of parts that prevent effective application of maximal force in the region being evaluated.

There is also a fundamental in the Fifth Edition of the AMA Guides, as well as all other Editions of the AMA Guides that are currently in use that one is to compare the unaffected joint when providing range of motion evaluations to establish a baseline and then rate the evaluated joint appropriately.

Concerning this, this lady would, therefore, have a 10 degree decrease from the contralateral side concerning flexion, a 25 degree decrease in extension, a 10 degree decrease in internal rotation, a 15 degree decrease in external rotation, a 20 degree decrease in abduction and no degree of decrease in adduction.

VALORIE GRANT
3/21/11
PAGE 7

Applying the appropriate values from Figures 16-40, 16-43 and 16-46 would then assign the following upper extremity percentage impairments to the right shoulder:

Flexion	1 percent
Extension	0 percent
Abduction	1 percent
Adduction	0 percent
Internal rotation	0 percent
External rotation	1 percent

According to the instructions in the Guides, these values are added together, as they are within the same joint, which would yield a 3 percent upper extremity impairment to the right shoulder. If administrative purposes dictate, this can be expressed as a 2 percent whole person impairment from Table 16-3 on page 439.

It is my opinion that this lady has reached a degree of maximum medical improvement for her right shoulder impingement syndrome condition.

Return to Work Issues

Concerning the issue of permanent recommendations for activity prescription concerning the right upper extremity, I would limit this lady's above shoulder-type of activities to only occasional. I would have no limitations concerning her left arm.

She would have no limitations as long as the work activities can be confined to an area from the belt line to the chest line. I believe it is inappropriate to assign any type of weight restriction concerning the right arm activities above shoulder use, but simply only limit the activity to an occasional basis.

Specific Questions

I have been asked several questions in a letter by Mr. Scheldrup dated March 16, 2011, which I respond to as follows:

1. "Do you believe the claimant's right shoulder condition and need for surgery are causally related to her work activity at Timmy's Catering or do you believe that it is more likely than not that claimant's right degenerative right condition and need for surgery are due to preexisting and/or nonindustrial medical condition and that her work at Timmy's Catering, while it may be one of the many factors, was not a substantial factor in bringing about her right shoulder condition and need for surgery?"

Answer: This is a very complex and compound sentence; however, I will answer it in its parts. First of all, based upon the evidence based medical literature that has been published on the subject of causation analysis for rotator cuff tendinitis and

VALORIE GRANT
3/21/11
PAGE 8

impingement syndrome, I am unable to identify the work activity at Timmy's Catering that would meet the threshold for that to be considered having causation, from the standpoint of the work activities.

The evidence based literature, on the other hand, would suggest that genetics and age play a larger role in the development of these problems.

It certainly would appear, based primarily on her diagnostic imaging, that this lady's shoulder impingement has developed, as it typically does in individuals over a number of years and on a continuum that has more to do with degeneration.

2. "If you believe claimant sustained a right shoulder injury as a result of her work activity at Timmy's Catering, do you believe that claimant sustained a permanent injury to her right shoulder as a result of his work activity at Timmy's Catering, or do you believe that claimant sustained, at most, a temporary exacerbation of a preexisting medical condition that returned to baseline?"

Answer: The answer is 'not applicable' as I do not believe that this right shoulder problem is a result of her work activity.

3. "Regardless of the causal mechanism of the same, when do you believe that claimant reached maximum medical improvement with regards to right shoulder injury?"

Answer: This would have occurred at some time after her surgical intervention. Typically after a decompression operation, this occurs somewhere between 8 and 12 weeks. It is somewhat difficult for me to pick a specific date, based upon the medical records that have been presented. I would simply give you that time reference framework as a reasoned, educated estimate.

4. "Regardless of the causal mechanism of the same, what permanent impairment, if any, would you assign for claimant's alleged right shoulder injury?"

Answer: The impairment rating for the right shoulder impingement syndrome condition is 3 percent of the upper extremity. Please see the Impairment section of the report above for a detailed description of the calculation of this, based upon the AMA Guides, Fifth Edition rules and protocols.

5. "Regardless of the causal mechanism of the same, what permanent restrictions, if any, would you assign the claimant's alleged right shoulder injury?"

Answer: I would limit her overhead activities with the right arm to only on an occasional basis.

6. "Regardless of the causal mechanism of the same, what future treatment, if any, would you recommend for claimant's shoulder ankle?"

Answer: I am unaware of any ankle condition, but I would not suggest that any additional treatment is required for her right shoulder condition.

VALORIE GRANT
3/21/11
PAGE 9

Conclusion

The above statements have been made with a reasonable degree of medical certainty/probability.

The opinions rendered in this case are the opinion of this evaluator. This evaluation has been conducted on the basis of medical examination and documentation as provided, with the expectation this material is true and correct. If more information becomes available at a later date, an additional service/report/reconsideration may be requested. Such information may or may not change the opinions rendered in this evaluation. This opinion is based on clinical assessment, examination and documentation. This opinion does not constitute, per se, recommendations for specific claims or administrative functions to be made or enforced.

If you have any questions with respect to this evaluation, please contact me personally through the office.

Sincerely,

Douglas W. Martin, MD, FACOEM, FAADEP, FAAFP, CIME, CEDIR

Fellow, American College of Occupational & Environmental Medicine
Fellow, American Academy of Disability Evaluating Physicians
Fellow, American Academy of Family Physicians
Certified Independent Medical Examiner (ABIME)
Certified Evaluator of Disability & Impairment Rating (AADEP)

DWM/lap

Appendix A

Medical Records Reviewed Valorie Grant

1. Medical records summary provided by Scheldrup Blades
2. Records from Krull Chiropractic Center
3. Medical records from Tri-State Orthopedics of Sioux City, Iowa
4. Records from Medical Associates Family Medicine Clinic of LeMars, Iowa
5. Medical records from Floyd Valley Hospital of LeMars, Iowa
6. Medical records from Siouxland Orthopedics and Sports Medicine Clinic, Sioux City, Iowa
7. Correspondence from Brian Johnson, M.D., Center for Neurosciences, Orthopedics and Spine, P.C.
8. Medical records from Northwest Surgery Associates
9. Additional medical records from Floyd Valley Hospital
10. Deposition transcript of Valorie Grant
11. Photograph of a motorcycle said to be claimant's husband's

November 7, 2016

TELMA LOUISE
PROGRAM SPECIALIST
NORTH NEBRASKA WORKFORCE SAFETY & INSURANCE
P.O. BOX 5585
LINCOLN, NE 66666

RE:	Lawrence Jughead
CLAIM#:	4569-878811
SS#:	XXX-XX-1045
DOB:	10/27/1947
DOI:	11/06/12

Dear Ms. Louise:

Please be advised that I had the opportunity to evaluate the above named individual at my office at 4230 War Eagle Drive in Sioux City, Iowa for purposes of an Independent Medical Examination for impairment rating derivation purposes on October 21, 2016.

Please be advised that the examinee read, understood and signed the notice of informed consent for Independent Medical Evaluation and this was placed in his chart. He was accompanied the entire time during the course of his history and physical examination by his wife.

Previously, he was earlier in the day seen by Steve Ferguson, O.D. for purposes of documenting visual field and visual acuity, as well as other visual issues which will be used for purposes of impairment derivation and will be included in this report.

Thank you for your introductory letter dated July 13, 2016. You have sent to me a CD of this gentleman's past medical records, which encompass 1,706 pages. For a list of the records reviewed by source, please see Appendix A attached to this report.

History of Present Illness

Mr. Lawrence Jughead is a 68-year-old white male who presents himself today for an Independent Medical Examination, at the request of North Nebraska Workforce Safety and Insurance Program Specialist, Telma Louise, to determine impairment rating with regards to conditions of left eye, cervical spine, and left hip abnormalities.

This gentleman states that he was involved in a commercial truck accident on November 6, 2012 in Arkansas. He, apparently, was drinking coffee and choked on it, which led him to veer off of the road, where he had a substantial impact trauma to the cab. Emergency medical personnel were dispatched to the scene and it took several hours for him to be extricated from the vehicle. He was subsequently taken to the Baptist Health Medical Center in Little Rock, Arkansas, where he was evaluated by trauma services. He had diagnostic testing that showed a left pedicle and pars fracture at the C6 level, as well as a nondisplaced linear fracture involving the left paramedian aspect of the anterior arch of C1. He was also noted to have

LAWRENCE JUGHEAD
11/07/16
PAGE 2

multilevel degenerative conditions of his cervical spine. He had a subdural hemorrhage that was not thought to need to have any type of immediate surgical attention. He had a left displaced orbital floor fracture with intrusion of the intraorbital fat and there was some degree of intraorbital hemorrhage that occurred. He also was noted to have an ocular laceration.

He was kept in the hospital for several days and eventually was discharged to home. There was definite identification of need to have surgical intervention regarding his ocular laceration. However, the physicians did not feel his orbital floor fracture was something that required immediate attention. After he got back to his home in Cherokee, Iowa, he saw his primary care physician, Dr. Veit and then subsequently other specialty physicians at the University of Iowa. He was treated in a collar for his cervical spine fractures and it was determined that he did not need to have any additional intervention for that. In discussion with him, he does not give any symptoms consistent with a radicular issue or problem.

He had some comorbid issues that he had to take care of regarding an abdominal aortic aneurysm and subsequently had to have a surgery for that, which was complicated by a Methicillin-resistant Staphylococcus aureus infection that required some additional surgical intervention. As he also carried a diagnosis of chronic obstructive pulmonary disease, coronary artery disease (which required previous stents) and Wolff-Parkinson-White arrhythmia, they were very careful to monitor him during this process. His orbital floor fracture was eventually operated on, but, unfortunately, he was left with issues regarding blurry vision and double vision, and those continue to be an issue for him today. He had previously been seen by Dr. Ferguson, who is an Optometrist affiliated in the Dakota Dunes area, for a variety of different strategies to try to help with this, including prism-type glasses.

He was under the care of Dr. Blow in Sioux Falls, South Dakota for rehabilitation needs and was sent to physical therapy to work on a variety of conditions, including neck pain and shoulder pain. After he had his physical therapy, he, unfortunately, continued to complain of neck pain and now also is complaining of lower back pain. The medical records would reflect that he also started to have issues with his left hip, which were evaluated by Orthopedic Surgeon, Dr. Hermanson in Sioux Falls, South Dakota. An MRI scan imaging study showed that there may have been a degree of labral abnormality, but it was felt that this was not necessarily due to trauma and Dr. Hermanson did not believe that there would necessarily be any help, from a surgical standpoint.

He has had multiple injections done by the Dakota Dunes Pain Clinic regarding back, hip and actually shoulder concerns.

More recently, he has been followed by Dr. Adams, who is a physician from Norfolk who comes up and does a clinic in South Sioux City. They have seen him

LAWRENCE JUGHEAD
11/07/16
PAGE 3

on multiple different occasions and he has had multiple different recommendations—some of which happened and others which have not. The wife expresses concern about intravenous treatments that he gets and is referring to Decadron and Toradol, and openly questions whether or not those treatments are reasonable and necessary.

In discussion with Mr. Jughead today, he states that his visual problems are the most paramount things that he has to deal with. He complains of neck stiffness, which, would not necessarily be surprising. But, again, he does not complain of any radiation in the arms that could be construed to have a dermatomal distribution. He does have some left shoulder discomfort which seems to be related to some degenerative issues there.

Regarding his left hip, he does have some come-and-go type of discomfort in that area, but he actually is complaining more of back pain to me today than anything. There does not appear to be any radicular phenomenon to his problem, but he does state that the problems seem to interfere with his walking activities, and he has a single cane that he uses in his right hand. Given the way that he walked around in the examination room, and the fact that he was also complaining to me of some balance issues, which probably are related to some of his vision trouble, I did ask if he had contemplated a walker, and they told me that he had a 4-pronged walker on order which has a seat, which I think would be an excellent alternative for him.

Review of Systems

His Review of Systems is positive for coronary artery disease, abdominal aortic aneurysm, chronic obstructive pulmonary disease, gastroesophageal reflux disease, and extremity edema.

Past Medical History

Current Medications: Include Tramadol 50 mg. q.i.d; Gabapentin 300 mg. that he takes anywhere from 4 to 8 times a day; Isosorbide Extended Release 30 mg. daily; Spironolactone 25 mg. daily; Atorvastatin 20 mg. daily; Furosemide 40 mg. daily; Pantoprazole 20 mg. daily; Trazodone 50 mg. daily; Venlafaxine 75 mg. daily; Montelukast 10 mg. q. day; Co-Q supplements; Vitamin D3 supplement; aspirin 81 mg. daily; Glucosamine Chondroitin supplement; Bupropion 150 mg. q. day; Hydrocodone/acetaminophen 7.5 mg./325, 1 q.i.d.

LAWRENCE JUGHEAD
11/07/16
PAGE 4

Allergies: He Has No Known Medical Allergies

Family History	: Positive for cancer and coronary artery disease.
Occupational History	: Reveals that he drove a commercial truck for greater than 30 years.
Social History	: Reveals that he currently smokes 5 cigarettes daily, down from a maximum of 2 packs a day in the past. He denies alcohol or illicit drug use.
Surgical History	: Positive for his left eye surgery, left shoulder rotator cuff surgery, a cholecystectomy, heart stent and abdominal stent placement that required a redo operation due to Methicillin-resistant Staphylococcus aureus infection development.

Physical Examination

The gentleman was pleasant and cooperative during the course of the history taking and physical examination. He walked into the examination room with utilization of a single cane that he used into his right hand, and it was noted that his gait pattern was antalgic. He was able to get in and out of the chair, and off and on the examination table with no assistance, but it took him extra time in order to accomplish that.

His visual appearance of his facial structures reveals that there is a visible abnormality and anophthalmos-type situation with regards to his left eye, no doubt from his orbital floor fracture. He has a tendency to not want to open his left eye because of issues that he is experiencing with respect to diplopia. His funduscopic examination and extraocular movement, as well as other visual function tests will be reported out by Dr. Ferguson in his notes. Otherwise, his cranial nerve examination is unremarkable.

The ear, nose and throat examination is unremarkable as well.

NECK : Supple. There is no lymphadenopathy or mass.

HEART: Regular rate and rhythm without murmur.

LUNGS: Reveal coarse breath sounds bilaterally.

Specific examination to his cervical spine shows that there is diffuse tenderness upon palpation of the paracervical structures. There is no evidence of any paravertebral muscle tone loss, atrophic change or spasm. His range of motion is grossly symmetrical. He is able to flex to 40 degrees, extend to 40 degrees, right and left laterally flex to 35 degrees, and right and left rotate to 60 degrees. Spurling's maneuver for

LAWRENCE JUGHEAD
11/07/16
PAGE 5

radiculopathy is not revealing. There is some crepitus with both active and passive motion of the cervical spine, consistent with some degenerative conditions. I do not see any evidence of occipital nerve abnormalities. Tinel's testing over both the greater and lesser occipital nerves are negative.

Examination of his left hip showed that he had diffuse complaints with range of motion. Palpably, there does not appear to be any substantial pain into the hip proper. However, there is discomfort upon palpation over the left lower paralumbar segments. No kyphosis or scoliosis are identified. He had some degree of discomfort also over the left sacroiliac joint. There is no paravertebral muscle tone loss, atrophic change or spasm of the lumbar spine identified.

His lower extremity reflexes of the patellae and Achilles are 2+ and symmetric. Light touch and two-point discrimination testing show a minor stocking glove distribution abnormality probably more consistent with peripheral vascular disease than anything. Indeed, after we removed his shoes and socks, there is a significant degree of ruddy cyanotic appearance to his feet and toes. I can not feel a dorsalis pedis or posterior tibial pulse. The strength of dorsiflexion, plantar flexion, quadriceps and hamstring strength are 5/5 and symmetric. I do not measure any degree of muscle tone loss or atrophy in either the quadriceps or the calf areas.

He certainly does have some end range of motion discomfort with regards to the left hip. But, there is also some of that in the right hip - although it is not as significant. The range of motion of the left hip shows that he is able to flex to 90 degrees, extend to 10 degrees, internally rotate to 20 degrees, externally rotate to 40 degrees, laterally abduct to 40 degrees and adduct to 20 degrees. This is largely symmetrical with the unaffected right hip area.

Finally, as we stated, his gait pattern was assessed. He has an antalgic gait pattern favoring his left leg. He utilizes a single cane in his right hand, which does help his ambulatory status, both from a speed and stability standpoint. We did not have him perform heel-toe or tandem gait secondary to these issues, nor did we have him attempt any squatting.

Assessment

1. History of traumatic brain injury with subdural hematoma; managed conservatively
2. Left orbital floor fracture; managed conservatively
3. Left eye abnormality secondary to #2 above with diplopia and visual difficulties
4. Cervical spine fracture of the pars and the facet at C6 and the arch at C1, nondisplaced; managed conservatively

LAWRENCE JUGHEAD
11/07/16
PAGE 6

5. Left hip injury, difficult to characterize; probably a sprain or a strain; I doubt, and would be in agreement with the Orthopedic Surgeon that the labral abnormality would not be necessarily traumatic in its origin
6. Degenerative disease of the lumbar spine
7. Degenerative disease of the cervical spine
8. History of chronic obstructive pulmonary disease
9. History of coronary artery disease
10. History of aneurysm, status post repair with infection complications
11. History of hypercholesterolemia
12. Peripheral vascular disease
13. Gastroesophageal reflux disease

Prognosis

This gentleman's prognosis is **fair**.

Recommendations

I have no additional medical care recommendations for Mr. Jughead regarding the injuries sustained as a result of his commercial motor vehicle accident.

Causation

Causation, in this case, is based upon review of the medical documentation as presented, as well as interview with the examinee. I do not think there is any question that this gentleman's motor vehicle accident created the 2 areas of the cervical spine fracture, as well as the left orbital floor fracture and residual visual problems that he has with his left eye thereafter.

Less clear is the situation with regards to his left hip. It is probably true that some degree of injury occurred. Whether this was a strain, a sprain, a bad contusion, some other soft tissue issue or what have you, is probably a more likely explanation as to what has occurred there. I would agree with the Orthopedic Surgeon that his labral abnormality would not necessarily be trauma related and probably is better explained by degenerative processes.

He has some degenerative issues with regards to his lumbar spine which seem to be fairly significant for him. However, I do not think that those things are trauma related.

LAWRENCE JUGHEAD
11/07/16
PAGE 7

He is not the most healthy person in the world, having had issues with chronic obstructive pulmonary disease, coronary artery disease, peripheral vascular disease and so forth. I think these comorbidities likely play a role with respect to perhaps slow or incomplete healing, with regards to some of his other trauma related issues.

Impairment

Impairment rating, in this case, is based upon the principles of the American Medical Association Guides to the Evaluation of Permanent Impairment, Sixth Edition, as well as the principles and practices and utilization of those Guides, as taught by the International Academy of Independent Medical Evaluators (previously known as the American Academy of Disability Evaluating Physicians) and as tested by that organization, as well as that by the American Board of Independent Medical Examiners.

This gentleman's left eye impairment rating, with regards to his impairment of visual field and visual acuity, is based upon the information obtained from Dr. Ferguson's office.

The results of visual acuity and visual field testing were obtained from Dr. Steven Ferguson's office on November 7, 2016.

The gentleman's visual acuity assessment was actually equal in both the left and the right eye with distance visual acuity of 20/25 OD and 20/25 OS.

Visual field score information was reviewed and the visual field test actually indicated that the gentleman had more of a visual field deficit in the right eye than he necessarily had in the left. There could be a variety of reasons for this, but probably is representative of other chronic medical condition issues. The point of this is that it does not appear that the trauma has affected the visual field independently any greater with regards to the left than what is included in the right eye.

In looking at this information and applying it to the Visual System, Chapter 12, in the AMA Guides, Sixth Edition, I do not think that one can necessarily apply an impairment rating due to the trauma, therefore, with regards to any type of visual field issue, per se, with the left eye.

Regarding the visual acuity situation, given the fact that the right and the left eye are equal at 20/25, I also do not think that one could assign an impairment rating to the injury with the left eye specifically.

I do believe, however, that the issue with regards to the gentleman's diplopia from his visual system would be appropriately identified. Diplopia is an adjustment to the visual impairment rating system evaluation, which is discussed within Section

LAWRENCE JUGHEAD
11/07/16
PAGE 8

12.4.b. beginning on page 305. Essentially, with regards to the instructions on page 306 in the first column, point #4, the issue here is with respect to assessing any interference with activities of daily living with regards to whatever extent suppression may reduce the awareness of double vision.

As indicated in the report above, Mr. Jughead has a tendency to keep his left eye closed to avoid any type of diplopia situation. I am not sure that I necessarily can state that it is so severe that it warrants continuous occlusion, as discussed in the AMA Guides, Sixth Edition. In that type of a situation, the impairment is suggested to be a 20 point loss. I think that it is probably more than just 1 quadrant. As is typically the case with regards to these orbital-type of blowout fractures, either the superior or inferior 2 quadrants are affected. Thus, I think that one-half of this value is probably the more appropriate way of looking at the true impact on activities of daily living.

As such, I would assign a 10 percent visual system impairment rating to the situation, with regards to the diplopia problems with respect to the left eye.

The visual system impairment of 10 percent equals a 10 percent whole person impairment.

The other issue dealing with his left eye problem is the fact of the visual abnormality with respect to the orbital floor fracture, which is visible on examination. One would need to take into consideration Chapter 11 of the Ear, Nose, Throat and Related Structures in order to determine any impairment from that. Appropriate application of Table 11-5 dealing with facial disorders/disfigurement would seem appropriate, especially given the criteria under Section 11.3 of the face, which begins on page 260.

In my opinion, this gentleman would best be categorized as a Class 2 level of impairment because the physical examination does show a loss of some of the supporting structures of the orbital floor and would include depressed appearance, with regards to his lower orbital areas. He does have x-ray studies that are consistent with this. Although he does not have any obstruction of the nasal passages and his shortness of breath probably is best described by his chronic obstructive pulmonary disease issues, I think that there is a strong argument that this Class is more appropriate than Class 1.

An 8 percent impairment of the whole person is afforded as a baseline for that particular Class. The determination with regards to varying from that Class is given within the instructions on page 261. Since the key factor is the History, the Physical Examination would also be a Class 2 level of descriptor. The diagnostic tests also would be a Class 2 level of descriptor. I think that the gentleman would, therefore, stay within the 8 percent whole person impairment rating for that particular condition.

LAWRENCE JUGHEAD
11/07/16
PAGE 9

Regarding his cervical spine fractures at the C1 arch and C6 pars and facets, this is assessed according to the Spine and Pelvis Chapter, with correspondence to the Cervical Spine Regional Grid.

This gentleman would be rated under Fractures/Dislocations of the Spine, as discussed within Table 17-2 and as described on page 565.

The determination of Class, in this particular situation, would seemingly be a decision between Class 0 and Class 1, as discussed within that Table. Class 0 is reserved for single or multiple fractures with minimal compression, which is appropriate in this situation, that have been healed with no residual signs or symptoms. Class 1 is reserved for single or multiple fractures that are healed with or without surgery, and an individual may have documented resolved radiculopathy or nonverifiable radicular complaints at clinically appropriate levels.

There has always been somewhat of an argument here as to whether or not that term "may" is a requirement or a necessity for the Class. But, in reality, it is not necessarily intended to be that. Thus, since the gentleman does have some degree of residual difficulty with respect to his neck, it would seemingly be most appropriate, I think, to place him in Class 1 simply from the standpoint that he has had fractures in 2 cervical levels - 1 at the C1 and 1 at the C6 level. Thus, I would choose Class 1 as his descriptor. Of course, the Grade C value with regards to that would be a 4 percent whole person impairment.

According to the Sixth Edition, adjustment factors need to be applied.

We had the gentleman complete the Pain Disability Questionnaire today, which is the identified methodology to determine the Grade Modifier for Functional History. This was scored at a 99.

According to Table 17-6 on page 575, this would yield a Grade Modifier 2 for Functional History.

Regarding the Physical Examination Grade Modifier, this is taken from Table 17-7 on page 576. This would be a Grade Modifier of 0.

The Grade Modifier for Clinical Studies is not applied, in this situation, because the diagnostic test of a CT scan documented the diagnosis. In that case, when a test is used to confirm or make the diagnosis, it is not applied as a Grade Modifier.

There is also another instruction in the AMA Guides here with regards to Grade Modifiers that is appropriate to be used, in that the Grade Modifier for Functional History is disregarded if it lies 2 or more levels different than either the Grade Modifiers for Physical Examination or Clinical Studies.

Thus, this gentleman's only Grade Modifier that is taken into consideration is for the Physical Examination, which I have said is 0. This would allow a Net Adjustment of −1, which would drop his impairment rating to the Grade B level within the Table

LAWRENCE JUGHEAD
11/07/16
PAGE 10

that was previously identified. Thus, his impairment rating for his cervical spine problem would be 2 percent of the whole person.

Regarding his left hip issue, this would be assessed utilizing the Lower Extremity Chapter, which is Chapter 16. Again, one would turn to the Diagnosis Regional Grid for the hip, which is within Table 16-4 beginning on page 512. I think that there could be an argument here to use an "other soft tissue lesion" as opposed to "strain." One could also look at the "acetabular or labral tear" on page 513. However, as we have previously indicated, we do not necessarily agree that the acetabular tear has any relationship to the trauma. Thus, one is challenged with using either the strain under the muscle tendon diagnosis, or the other soft tissue lesion area under the soft tissue diagnosis.

In actuality, it does not make any difference because one would pick the lower description value within each diagnosis. The gentleman does not have any motion deficits in his left hip that can be identified to be any different above and beyond the right hip, as we have indicated. Therefore, the palpatory and/or radiographic findings appear to be most appropriate to use here. That Default Grade C value is 1 percent of the lower extremity.

We do go through the process, again, of assigning the Grade Modifiers. In this case, for the Grade Modifier for Functional History, we had the gentleman complete the AAOS Lower Limb Questionnaire. Scoring this indicates that his standardized mean score is 47. His normative score is 18. This is indicative of a moderate problem, which would be assigned a Grade Modifier of 2.

Regarding his Physical Examination Adjustment from Table 16-7, he is probably best assigned to a Grade Modifier 1 for his minimal palpatory findings.

The Clinical Studies Adjustment from Table 16-8 is best termed as a Grade Modifier 0 because there are no relevant abnormalities that are found on the exam specific to the injury at hand.

Therefore, using the Net Adjustment Formula, one, again, is faced with having to disregard the Functional History Grade Modifier because it lies 2 or more values from the Grade Modifier for either the Physical Examination or the Clinical Studies. If one were to then use the Net Adjustment Formula, you would find that this would be a −1, which would, again, drop this down to a Grade B level of impairment and, going back into the Regional Grid for the hip, regarding the strain or the other soft tissue lesion area, this would still be at a 1 percent lower extremity impairment.

The 1 percent lower extremity impairment would need to be converted to a whole person impairment. This would also be a 1 percent whole person impairment (the conversion factor is 40 percent, but impairment ratings that are greater than absolute 0, but less than 0.5, are not rounded to 0, but, instead, are rounded up to 1).

Thus, this gentleman's final impairment rating would be a combination of the 8 percent whole person impairment from the facial disfigurement coupled with the 1 percent whole person impairment from the left hip injury, combined with the 10 percent impairment of the whole person to the visual system.

LAWRENCE JUGHEAD
11/07/16
PAGE 11

When one performs this function utilizing the Combined Values Table, this yields an 18 percent whole person permanent partial impairment rating.

The gentleman has reached a degree of maximum medical improvement.

Conclusion

The above statements have been made with a reasonable degree of medical certainty/probability.

The opinions rendered in this case are the opinion of this evaluator. This evaluation has been conducted on the basis of a medical examination and documentation as provided, with the expectation this material is true and correct. If more information becomes available at a later date, an additional service/report/reconsideration may be requested. Such information may or may not change the opinions rendered in this evaluation. This opinion is based on a clinical assessment, examination and documentation. This opinion does not constitute, per se, recommendations for specific claims or administrative functions to be made or enforced.

If you have any questions with respect to this evaluation, please contact me personally through the office.

Sincerely,

Douglas W. Martin, MD, FACOEM, FAADEP, FAAFP, CIME, CEDIR
Fellow, American College of Occupational & Environmental Medicine
Fellow, American Academy of Disability Evaluating Physicians
Fellow, American Academy of Family Physicians
Certified Independent Medical Examiner (ABIME)
Certified Evaluator of Disability & Impairment Rating (AADEP)

DWM/lap

TIME SPENT ON CONDUCTING HISTORY AND PHYSICAL EXAMINATION = 1-1/2 HOURS

TIME SPENT ON REVIEW OF MEDICAL RECORD DOCUMENTATION = 4 HOURS

TIME SPENT ON REPORT GENERATION, INCLUDING INCORPORATION
OF DR. FERGUSON'S INFORMATION,
REVIEW AND EDITING = 1 HOUR

Appendix A

Records Reviewed Lawrence Jughead

1. Medical records from the Baptist Health Medical Center of Little Rock, Arkansas
2. Various different care plan and correspondence issues surrounding that hospitalization
3. Medical records from Stephen Veit, M.D., Cherokee, Iowa
4. Sanford Health Clinic records, Sioux Falls, South Dakota, multiple providers
5. GENEX case management nursing correspondence from Mary Griffith, RN, BSN
6. Medical records from the University Hospital and Clinics, Oculoplastic Service
7. Other correspondence from the University Hospital and Clinics
8. Medical record information from the Cherokee Regional Medical Center of Cherokee, Iowa
9. Medical records from Jerry Blow, M.D., Sioux Falls Rehabilitation Specialists
10. Physical therapy notes from the Cherokee Regional Medical Center of Cherokee, Iowa
11. Medical records from Eli Chesen, M.D., Psychiatric Services of Lincoln
12. Medical records from Avera McKennan Hospital, Sioux Falls, South Dakota
13. Medical records from the Orthopedic Institute, Sioux Falls, South Dakota Evan Hermanson, M.D.
14. Medical records from Jeffrey Sykes, M.D., Cardiovascular Associates of Sioux City, Iowa
15. Medical records from the University of Iowa Hospital and Clinics, Neuro-Ophthalmological Service
16. Medical records from Siouxland Surgery Center Pain Clinic, Dakota Dunes, South Dakota
17. Medical records from Steve Ferguson, O.D., Dunes Eye Care
18. Neuropsychological evaluation, Neuropsychology Consultants, L.L.C., Michael McGraff, PhD, Sioux Falls, South Dakota
19. Functional Capacity Examination Report, Human Performance Testing's, Terry Nelson, P.T.
20. Report of Integrity Physical Therapy, Storm Lake, Iowa
21. Medical records from C. Robert Adams, M.D., Norfolk, Nebraska

SSDI IME Reports

ST. LUKE'S OCCUPATIONAL MEDICAL CLINIC
224 NORTH DERBY LANE
NORTH SIOUX CITY, SD 57049

NAME: Steven Certain
SS#: 615-46-4419
DATE: 1/02/07
DOB: 5/13/1991

STATE OF IOWA DISABILITY DETERMINATION SERVICES BUREAU
COMPREHENSIVE EXAMINATION REPORT

CHIEF COMPLAINT: Behavioral disorder, and right arm problems.

HISTORY OF PRESENT ILLNESS: This is a 15-year-old male who presents himself today at the request of the State of Iowa Disability Determination Services Bureau for comprehensive examination and report.

He is the product of an extremely difficult family situation. The gentleman has been a resident of a boy's ranch for trouble youth for a number of years. Apparently, his parents are basically out of the scene. He is currently being cared for by his uncle, who accompanies him in the examination room today.

The main problem that the gentleman has is with respect to behavioral disorders. He has been given the diagnosis of Attention Deficit Hyperactivity Disorder and his uncle relates that he has also been given the diagnosis of depression and schizophrenia in the past. He has difficulty with school work, concentration and other behavioral issues. There is a strong history of child abuse by the parents in the past. He has had multiple attempts of trying to attend regular school, but that has failed and he now goes to the Boys and Girls Home for individualized schooling.

He is on a number of psychiatric medications which the uncle tells me are going to need to be adjusted. He tells me that they have an appointment with a psychiatrist later today, as he is having difficulty maintaining behavioral control with the medications that he currently is taking.

From a medical standpoint, the gentleman had a forearm fracture approximately 1-1/2 years ago that was pinned and plated. He indicates that will occasionally give him some discomfort with activity, but he tells me that he is involved in training for ultimate fighting type of matches. This tells me that he actually is quite functional with it.

In addition, the gentleman states that he has a problem with asthma, which has been present for a number of years. He discusses difficulty with dyspnea on exertion and shortness of breath with extreme activity, but, again, as he is in the middle of training for these ultimate fighting type of activities, I would find it difficult to believe that it is significantly limiting to him.

REVIEW OF SYSTEMS: Except for that described above, is negative.

SURGICAL HISTORY: Positive for the right forearm open reduction and internal fixation.

CURRENT MEDICATIONS: Include DDAVP .2 mg., 2 q. h.s; Zyprexa inhaler q. 6 hours p.r.n; Risperdal 2 mg. q. h.s; Mirtazapine 15 mg. q. h.s; Zoloft 100 mg., 2 q. h.s; Hydroxyzine 25 mg. q. h.s; Singulair 10 mg. q. h.s; Concerta 36 mg., 2 q. a.m.

STEVEN CERTAIN
1/02/07
PAGE 2

Allergies: He Has No Known Medical Allergies

FAMILY HISTORY: Positive for cancer, coronary artery disease, diabetes mellitus.

SOCIAL HISTORY: Reveals that he is the product of significant problems with family violence and a distorted family situation in the past. He denies smoking, alcohol or illicit drug use.

OCCUPATIONAL/SCHOOL HISTORY: Reveals that he currently attends the Boys and Girls Home for high school.

PHYSICAL EXAMINATION: Height without shoes is 70.5″; weight is 261 pounds; blood pressure is 118/92; temperature is 98F; pulse is 80; respiratory rate is 18.

VISUAL ACUITY: Snellen equivalence at 20′ with corrective lenses, OD 20/30, OS 20/25; OU 20/25.

GENERAL APPEARANCE: Reveals a teenage boy who appears his stated age. He has a mohawk haircut. He sits on the examination table in an extremely forward, slouched type of posture.

HEENT: Reveals the head to be normocephalic. Eyes: Pupils equal, round, react to light and accommodation. Extraocular movements are intact. Normal funduscopic and normal conjunctival examination. The ear, nose and throat examination is positive for ceruminosis in the canals bilaterally, but otherwise benign.

NECK: Supple. There is no lymphadenopathy or mass.

HEART: Regular rate and rhythm without murmur.

LUNGS: Clear to auscultation and percussion.

ABDOMEN: Benign.

EXTREMITIES: Extremity examination reveals that the range of motion of the spine and extremities are as included in the enclosed range of motion form.

The right upper extremity reveals that there is an approximately 15 centimeter scar located over the volar surface of the mid portion of the right forearm, presumably in the area of the prior internal fixation. It is mildly tender upon palpation, but does not appear to negatively inhibit the wrist or elbow capabilities.

The strength of the bilateral rotator cuff musculature, biceps, triceps, wrist deviators and grip strength are 5/5 and symmetric. There is no muscular tone loss, atrophic change or spasm identified. Light touch and two-point discrimination testing are well within normal limits.

Examination of the cervical, thoracic and lumbar spines are without abnormality.

Lower extremity examination reveals normality with respect to the hips, knees, ankles and muscular tone loss is not appreciated. His strength is 5/5 throughout. Neurosensory examination is normal. Reflexes of the biceps, brachioradialis, triceps, patellae and Achilles are 1+ and symmetric.

Further neurologic examination reveals cranial nerves II-XII to be grossly intact. Rapid alternating movements are well within normal limits. He is able to perform heel-toe and tandem gait without difficulty. He is able to squat without difficulty.

STEVEN CERTAIN
1/02/07
PAGE 3

Assessment

1. Various psychological and psychiatric disorders including Attention Deficit Hyperactivity Disorder, history of depression, schizophrenia, behavioral and conduct disorders
2. History of right forearm fracture requiring open reduction and internal fixation
3. Asthma

Recommendations

With respect to this gentleman's remaining functional capacities, by far the issues with his psychological and psychiatric issues outweigh any problems from a physical nature. I do not think there are any limitations that I would place on him, from the standpoint of his right forearm or from his asthma. They appear to be under reasonably good control. With his activity level that he describes, I can not envision that his asthma would be limiting.

Therefore, I would have no concerns with respect to lifting, carrying, standing, moving about, walking, or sitting; nor would I have concerns with stooping, climbing, kneeling or crawling activities. I would have no issues with handling objects, seeing, hearing, speaking, traveling, or with issues concerning exposures to the work environment such as to dust, fumes, temperatures or hazards.

Obviously, I will let other professionals better able to comment on the psychiatric component of his claim for disability to comment upon such. Please find enclosed, for your review, the range of motion form. If you have any concerns or questions with respect to this examination, please do not hesitate to contact me.

Sincerely,

Douglas W. Martin, MD, FAADEP, FACOEM, FAAFP, CIME, CEDIR
Fellow, American Academy of Disability Evaluating Physicians
Fellow, American College of Occupational and Environmental Medicine
Fellow, American Academy of Family Physicians
Certified Independent Medical Examiner by the American Board of Independent Medical Examiners
Certified Evaluator of Disability and Impairment Rating

Medical License Number:	28886	(IA)	Exp.	03/01/07
	3939	(SD)	Exp.	02/28/07
	18932	(NE)	Exp.	10/01/08

DWM/lap

Enclosure

ST. LUKE'S OCCUPATIONAL MEDICAL CLINIC
224 NORTH DERBY LANE
NORTH SIOUX CITY, SD 57049

NAME: Carley Snowball
SS#: 320-52-4353
DATE: 1/04/07
DOB: 12/25/1953

STATE OF NEBRASKA DISABILITY DETERMINATION SERVICES BUREAU
COMPREHENSIVE EXAMINATION REPORT

CHIEF COMPLAINT: Sleep apnea problems, kidney trouble, and obesity.

HISTORY OF PRESENT ILLNESS: This is a 53-year-old Native American female who presents herself today at the request of the State of Nebraska Disability Determination Services Bureau for comprehensive examination and report.

This lady has been given a diagnosis of interstitial cystitis. She states that she has frequent bladder spasms and painful urination with frequent urinary tract infections. She, apparently, has been seen by renal specialists.

In addition to this, she has trouble with sleep apnea. She currently has a CPAP mask, which she is working with.

She complains of day time fatigue. Apparently, someone has discussed with her the possibility of fibromyalgia as a diagnosis; but, of course, this is difficult to assess, given her sleep apnea history. She does complain of neck and back pain, and difficulty going up and down stairs.

REVIEW OF SYSTEMS: Also positive for asthma and being deaf in the left ear (She states that this occurred as a result of childhood injury at age 10.). She also has a history of depression.

CURRENT MEDICATIONS: Include Cymbalta 30 mg. q. day; aspirin q. day; Elavil 10 mg. q. h.s; Albuterol inhaler 2 times a day; Allegra q. day; Singulair daily.

Allergies: She Has Stated Allergies To Penicillin And Latex

SURGICAL HISTORY: Positive for a right knee anterior cruciate ligament repair, cholecystectomy, tubal ligation, ganglion cyst removal of the right wrist, and right sided bunionectomy.

FAMILY HISTORY: Positive for cerebrovascular accident and diabetes mellitus.

SOCIAL HISTORY: Reveals that she does not smoke, abuse alcohol or use illicit drugs.

OCCUPATIONAL HISTORY: Reveals that she last worked as a social service worker.

PHYSICAL EXAMINATION: Height without shoes is 65-1/4″; weight is 277.6 pounds; blood pressure is 142/92; temperature is 98.4F; pulse is 84; respiratory rate is 18.

VISUAL ACUITY: Snellen equivalence at 20′ with contact lenses, OD 20/20, OS 20/25; OU 20/20.

CARLEY SNOWBALL
1/04/07
PAGE 2

HEENT: Reveals the head to be normocephalic. Eyes: Pupils equal, round, react to light and accommodation. Extraocular muscles are intact. Normal funduscopic and normal conjunctival examination. The ear, nose and throat examination is unremarkable.

NECK: Supple. There is no lymphadenopathy or mass.

HEART: Regular rate and rhythm without murmur.

LUNGS: Clear to auscultation and percussion.

ABDOMEN: Reveals diffuse tenderness over the superpubic area, but no rebound, guarding or masses appreciated. Bowel sounds are positive x 4 quadrants.

EXTREMITIES: The upper extremity examination reveals that the reflexes of the upper and lower extremities are 2+ and symmetric. The strength of major muscle group testing of both the upper and lower extremities are 5/5 throughout. There is no muscular tone loss, atrophic change or spasm identified.

Neurologic examination reveals that light touch and two-point discrimination testing are well within normal limits. I do not appreciate any significant limitations of any of the joints.

I did perform a tender point examination, per the American College of Rheumatology criteria. She had no positive tender points today in any of the 18 areas.

Further neurologic examination reveals cranial nerves II-XII to be grossly intact. Rapid alternating movements are well within normal limits. She is able to perform heel-toe and tandem gait and able to squat with some complaints of right knee pain.

Assessment

1. Obesity
2. Sleep apnea
3. History of asthma
4. Interstitial cystitis
5. Day time fatigue; etiology unclear
6. Deafness in the left ear from childhood injury
7. Mild residual knee pain from anterior cruciate ligament repair

Recommendations

With respect to this lady's remaining functional capabilities, I would first state that she had no difficulty understanding my speech at a normal volume, and I had no difficulty understanding her speech.

CARLEY SNOWBALL
1/04/07
PAGE 3

With respect to her orthopedic issues, she has some mild residual trouble from her right knee from an anterior cruciate ligament repair.

She is dealing with obesity and depression.

From the standpoint of impact on lifting and carrying, I would expect her to be able to perform between 25 and 30 pounds occasionally, 15 to 20 pounds frequently, and 5 to 10 pounds constantly.

With respect to standing, moving about, walking or sitting, I would have no particular concerns.

Stooping, climbing, kneeling and crawling activities would best be limited to about half of what would be considered normal.

With respect to handling objects, seeing, hearing, speaking, or traveling, I would have no particular concerns.

With respect to exposures in the work environment such as to dust, fumes, temperatures or hazards, I would have no particular issues.

As always, I will leave her remaining functional capacities to your current guidelines. If you have any concerns or questions with respect to this examination, please do not hesitate to contact me.

Sincerely,

Douglas W. Martin, MD, FAADEP, FACOEM, FAAFP, CIME, CEDIR
Fellow, American Academy of Disability Evaluating Physicians
Fellow, American College of Occupational and Environmental Medicine
Fellow, American Academy of Family Physicians
Certified Independent Medical Examiner by the American Board of Independent Medical Examiners
Certified Evaluator of Disability and Impairment Rating

Medical License Number:	28886	(IA)	Exp.	03/01/07
	3939	(SD)	Exp.	02/28/07
	18932	(NE)	Exp.	10/01/08

DWM/lap

Appendix 3: Exercise—Before and After Report Example

Before Example

Date

Managed Care Organization
Attn: Case Manager
Address
City, State Zip Code

Claimant:	Ms. XXXX
BWC Number:	
Date of Injury:	
Social Security Number:	
Employer:	THE COMPANY
Allowed Conditions:	Right Lateral Epicondylitis

Dear Case Manager:

At your request, I performed an independent medical examination on Ms. XXXX on November 15, 2XXX. It was explained to Ms. XXXX that the purpose of this examination was for evaluation purposes only and that no treatment would be undertaken. It was further explained to her that the client requesting and paying for the assessment would receive a report. Lastly, it was explained to Ms. XXXX that no medical relationship would be formed; thus no physician-patient relationship would be established during the course of this assessment.

A request is being made for an additional allowance of right carpal tunnel syndrome

CHIEF COMPLAINT: Hand pain and numbness.

HISTORY OF PRESENT ILLNESS: The following narrative was told to the examiner by Ms. XXXX and was dictated in her presence.

Ms. XXXX denied having an prior history of neck, upper back, shoulder, or upper extremity problems before 19XX. MS. XXXX worked intermittently for THE COMPANY since approximately 19XX. In 19XX she was rehired and worked at THE COMPANY continuously until 19XX. THE COMPANY is now known as THE COMPANY. MS. XXXX worked as an equipment technician, where she ran a bender and/or saws. She stated that the bender machine did not run properly. She said when operating the bender, she would slide parts for framing windows. In the spring of 19XX the machine jerked and caused her to jerk her right arm. She stated that she quickly had right lateral elbow swelling and pain, but that her entire arm also hurt. She was initially diagnosed as having tennis elbow. X-rays were performed. She was told to use a forearm or (tennis elbow) band. She had injections over a period of several visits. At this point in time she was seeing her family doctor, but continued to work, usually seven days a week.

Ms. XXXX indicated that her elbow and arm continued to bother her, especially her shoulder. She complained of having shoulder pain at night, which would wake her. She stated that placing her shoulder and arm in a sling type position seemed to help decrease the discomfort. Once every other week, the pain in her right shoulder would become excruciating, at which time the pain would radiate into the right arm to the elbow. Using ice seemed to help, sometimes. The pain in the shoulder was so severe at times that she was unable to go to work.

One morning some time in mid to late October 19XX, she could not use her shoulder because of severe pain and swelling. She thought that the last day she worked was October 13, 19XX. She followed up with Dr. K at her family physician's office, who referred her to an orthopedic surgeon, Dr. D. An arthrogram was subsequently performed and a tear in the right rotator cuff was found. She had surgery to repair the right rotator cuff in December 19XX (surgery had been delayed secondary to problems with her asthma and chronic bronchitis).

Ms. XXXX stated that she has had significant pain since before and after having surgery to her right shoulder. She stated the pain has not improved since surgery, but does wax and wane in severity. She attended six weeks of physical therapy at HHHH HOSPITAL and then eight additional weeks performing work hardening at CCCC CENTERr. She underwent several nerve blocks, which relieved the pain only briefly. She also spent six weeks in the pain program at THE CENTER in Columbus, Ohio. She finished that program in September 19XX. She stated that the program did not help relieve her pain.

She has pain when lying on her shoulder, at night the pain wakes her up. She has severe pain approximately once a month. She had no improvement in shoulder movement after surgery. The severity of the shoulder pain varies significantly. She can be moderately pain free at rest. Using ice does help. Reaching forward is less bothersome than reaching laterally. Reaching behind her is especially bothersome. She occasionally gets neck and right upper back pain and spasms. Pain worsens with lifting, such that she can no longer lift a one gallon jug of milk. She has difficulty getting groceries out of her car. She has markedly decreased activities of daily living such as house cleaning, because of the shoulder pain and right upper extremity weakness. She now has to get help performing her normal housekeeping chores. She had decreased sleep secondary to her shoulder problem, but it has worsened because of her recent hand difficulties.

She stated that she has been on Social Security Disability since 19XX. She is unable to lift like she used to. She is also unable to perform repetitive activities using her shoulders. Her right shoulder strength is markedly decreased. She stated that her right elbow has not been treated or evaluated since 19XX. The right elbow pain is not as severe as it was initially after the accident. The right elbow can be pain free for several days in a row. The right elbow can be exacerbated with lifting type activities and can be painful for several days in a row. She believes her right elbow has some swelling in it on a fairly persistent basis. She wears a forearm band which does seem to help when she has to lift.

She has had some right hand or other upper extremity difficulties for the past 9–12 months. Her right hand, including all digits and the thumb, can go numb. This can occur during the day, but especially happens at night. It can wake her several times a night and the numbness can be present when she wakes up in the morning. She also noted that she has recurrent right hand swelling. She noted that this numbness can last for a while. She said because of her right upper extremity difficulties she has been using her left hand more (especially since the shoulder injury). She denied having any left handed numbness, but she has had pain at the ulnar side of the left wrist and hand for several months.

Dr. D has been evaluating her for her upper extremity difficulties and had wanted to do electrodiagnostic testing of the right upper extremity. This was not completed until May 2XXX, when testing by Dr. H demonstrated right carpal tunnel syndrome. Dr. D advised her to undergo carpal tunnel release, but she is not certain if she wants this performed. She has been dropping objects with both hands. She has recurrent hand swelling, the right usually worse than the left. The left has been bothering her more recently. She uses a wrist splint on the right side at night which helps decrease her symptoms. She also uses a left wrist band, which helps support her left wrist.

She recently lifted a jewelry box, maybe 5 pounds in weight, with her left hand. She ended up dropping the box. It twisted her left wrist, which increased her left wrist pain. She specifically denied ever having any injuries to her upper extremities since 1996. As part of this claim, she stated that she has been seen for both depression and anxiety. She has been treated by a psychologist for this condition.

She denied having any testing for thyroid, arthritis, or diabetes. She stated that she has had a 20-30 pound weight loss over the past year. She complained of having decreased weight, decreased sleep, decreased appetite, but denied having any fevers. She stated that she has nocturia, which has increased recently, although she indicated that she has also increased her fluid intake recently.

During the discussion with Ms. XXXX regarding the development of her symptoms, she persistently reiterated that she had no problems with her hands until after she had injured her right upper extremity. She noted that she has had a gradual onset of bilateral hand and wrist symptoms over the past several years. She specifically denied any new incident or injury to her upper extremities during this time frame. Over the past year, she has been less able to extend her fingers. This has worsened to the point where she is no longer able to fully extend certain fingers of both hands. Her hands are very stiff in the morning. This can last easily for half an hour or longer. She stated that some mornings she has to pry her fingers open. She complained of having ongoing finger pain and stiffness, as well as wrist pain and stiffness. She has recurrent swelling in her distal upper extremities, primarily involving the hands and fingers. She reiterated that her right hand is worse than her left, but that the left has very similar if not identical symptoms to the right, except for the lack of tingling and numbness.

PAST MEDICAL HISTORY: Ms. XXXX has undergone the following surgeries: surgical repair of her right earlobe, 19XX; hysterectomy, bilateral salpingo-oophorectomy, and appendectomy, 19XX; low back surgery (L3-4, L4-5) with residual left leg symptoms from nerve damage, 19XX; and right rotator cuff repair, 19XX. She has been hospitalized for hemoptysis, 19XX and for hypertension, 19XX. Other past medical problems have included a history of sinus and allergy problems since 19XX; diagnosis of irritable bowel syndrome in 19XX; history of recurrent bladder infections; a history of gastric ulcers times two, 19XX or 19XX, also associated with gastritis and accompanying esophageal stricture, status post dilation. She also was diagnosed with hypertension, 19XX; diagnosed with asthma, 19XX; diagnosed with coronary artery disease with a 50% posterior coronary block, 19XX; and diagnosed with depression and anxiety, 19XX. Past musculoskeletal problems include a removal of a ganglionic cyst from her right hand in the 19XXs, the low back injury with resultant surgery in 19XX, diagnosis of left knee bursitis requiring drainage in 19XX, the diagnosis of tennis elbow in 19XX, the right rotator cuff tear and rotator cuff repair in 19XX, diagnosis of right shoulder tendonitis, 19XX; diagnosis of right forearm tendonitis, 2XXX and diagnosis of carpal tunnel syndrome, 2XXX. Medications include Prilosec, Ultram, Soma compound, Elavil, Allegra, Tenormin, Albuterol, Singulair, Flovent, Seravent, Estratab, and an aspirin a day. She denied having any allergies to medications.

FAMILY HISTORY: There is a family history of high blood pressure, heart attack, stroke, bleeding problems, ulcers, obesity, birth defects, diabetes, cerebral palsy, asbestosis and cancer. Her father is deceased at the age of __ years from asbestos disease and cancer. Her mother is alive and well at the age of __ years. She has ____ brothers, ages ______ who are all alive and well, except that the oldest and youngest both have diabetes. She has ____ living children, ages_______. A sixth child was born with cerebral palsy and died in 19XX. She is currently divorced from her only marriage.

SOCIAL HISTORY: She has not smoked in 5–6 years, but does have a 15–20 pack year smoking history. She does not consume alcohol and denied recreational drug use. She does enjoy reading, primarily the bible. She occasionally plays card games or checkers with her grandchildren. She denied performing any repetitive hand activities as far as hobbies. She denied performing any regular exercise, although she does try to walk once a week. She has no pets at home. She wears glasses.

OCCUPATIONAL HISTORY: Ms. XXXX worked at ANOTHER COMPANY in SOMEPLACE, Ohio from 19XX – 19XX doing spot welding on an automatic sealer. After that she worked at ANOTHER PLACE cleaning offices from 19XX – 19XX. She also worked at A NURSING HOME as a nursing assistant from 19XX – 19XX. She worked continuously at THE COMPANY (formerly THE COMPANY) from 19XX – 19XX, and also worked there previously on an intermittent basis and during lay-offs she worked at nursing homes.

She has had past occupational exposures to grinding dust, metal dust, other dust, engine exhaust, smoke, other fumes mists or vapors, ammonia, welding fumes, acids and/or caustics, oils, metal coolants, viruses, noise, cold, heavy lifting, change in shift work, repetitive mechanical work and poor lighting.

REVIEW OF SYSTEMS: She is a gravida X, para X, with X living children. She has a history of bleeding problems. There is a history of hemophilia in the family. She has trouble sleeping. She has intermittently blurry vision. She has persistent ringing in her ears since 19XX. She has a history of sinus problems. She has a history of cough, some shortness of breath at rest, recurrent wheezing and congestion. She has coughed up blood in the past, including while at work in 19XX-19XX. She has a history of chest pain, but this has been less since resuming female replacement hormones. She also has a history of heart flutter and a history of high blood pressure. She complains of having a change of appetite and of having heart burn. She does get up a lot at night to urinate. She has complaints of anxiety, depression, confusion, and memory problems. She has a history of pain, swelling, or stiffness in her joints, arthritis, pain or numbness in her extremities, of having muscle cramps, of having low back pain or stiffness, of having neck pain or stiffness, of having swelling in her ankles, and of having some joint deformities and decreased function.

PAIN ASSESSMENT: On the Borg's pain scale, she rated her current pain as a 5. On the Borg's pain scale, 0 is no pain at all and 10 is a very very strong pain. She indicated that over the past 30 days her best level of pain was a level 5 and at it's worst it was a level 8. She stated that she is more limited by her hand movements than the pain. With further questioning, she noted that she did not get pain in the tip of her tailbone, that her whole leg does not become painful, nor does it go numb, nor does it give away. She did indicate that she has not had any spells with very little pain during the past year. These answers were not the same as those when she initially answered the questionnaire. On the Visual Analogue Pain Scale, she marked near the 50% mark, which correlates with her responses on the Borg's Analogue Pain Scale. Her responses on the McGill Pain Questionnaire totaled 33, which demonstrates a tendency to abnormal psychodynamics. Her responses on the Ransford Pain Drawing are consistent with the stated complaints. Ms. XXXX's responses using the pain assessment tools do not indicate significant pain symptom magnification, but are not entirely normal.

PHYSICAL EXAMINATION: This was a well-developed, well-nourished right hand dominant over weight 54 year old black female with short black hair and glasses. Her vital signs were all normal except for mildly elevated blood pressure at 152/96. Her height was 5′ 6½″ tall. Her weight was 217 pounds. Although she was pleasant and cooperative throughout the interview process and during the examination, her responses seemed somewhat delayed. Her affect appeared flat. In general, she appeared to be somewhat depressed.

She ambulated somewhat slowly with a wide based gait and a slight limp. Neck range of motion was mildly decreased, especially left lateral bending. No guarding was observed during active neck range of motion. There was no pain elicited with gentle cervical compression. No masses were palpated in the neck. There was posterior cervical paraspinal muscle tenderness palpated especially at both occiputs, as well as point tenderness of the central right cervical paraspinal muscles. There was tenderness to palpation of the right rhomboid, right trapezius, and right infraspinatus muscles. There was no tenderness to palpation of the cervical or thoracic spine. Back range of motion was fair with some decreased anterior flexion and lateral bending. No scapular winging was appreciated. A well healed lower mid-line surgical back scar was visualized.

Multiple tender points were palpated including over the left greater trochanter, left buttock, both trapezius muscles, at the occiputs bilaterally, both rhomboids, at the right anterior chest, right deltoid, and right dorsal forearm. A well-healed surgical scar was visualized over the anterior portion of the right shoulder. Active shoulder range of motion revealed the following: right shoulder abduction was 80° while left shoulder abduction was 120° (normal being 170°+). Right shoulder adduction was 10° while left shoulder adduction was 30° (normal being 50°). Right shoulder flexion was 90° while left shoulder flexion was 135° (normal being 180°). At 90° of abduction (somewhat less on the right), left external and internal rotation reached 45°, (normal internal rotation being 80° or greater, and external rotation being 60° or greater). Right internal shoulder rotation at approximately 80° of shoulder abduction, reached 35° with the above normals previously being described. No right shoulder external rotation was elicited. No shoulder laxity was elicited. There was tenderness to palpation of the right anterior chest, throughout the right glenohumeral joint, the right acromioclavicular joint and right deltoid. The anterior chest and deltoid tenderness was limited to point tenderness. There was no right arm or clavicle tenderness to palpation. No obvious swelling, deformity, or atrophy was appreciated, except at the hands. There was marked decreased strength of the right shoulder and was associated with give way weakness.

A well healed scar was visualized on the left dorsal radial wrist. There was tenderness to palpation of the left wrist, at the anatomic stuff box, and of the left hand, especially at the metacarpal phalangeal joints, and over the second through fifth proximal interphalangeal (PIP) finger joints. This tenderness was slightly less over the third PIP. There was also slight discomfort to palpation at the left distal interphalangeal finger joints. There was some slight swelling throughout the hands and wrists primarily over the metacarpal phalangeal joints and fingers. No thenar atrophy was appreciated. There was also tenderness to palpation over the right wrist, right anatomic stuff box, and over the right metacarpal phalangeal finger joints and second and third proximal interphalangeal finger joints. The right hand swelling was similar to that of the left. She complained of mildly decreased sensation throughout the fingers and thumb of the right hand, especially over the thumb, third and second digits. She had markedly decreased grip strength bilaterally. She also had markedly decreased opposition of her thumb with the fourth and fifth fingers, especially on the right. No crepitus was appreciated of either upper extremity. There was decreased supination bilaterally and decreased wrist flexion and extension, especially on the left. Finklestein's maneuver elicited no symptoms bilaterally. Elbow flexion appeared to be mildly decreased but was symmetrical, with decreased elbow extension, the right reaching 160° while the left reaching 170° (normal being 180°). There was tenderness to palpation of the right lateral epicondyle and into the adjacent dorsal forearm, but not at the olecranon or antecubital fossa. Pulses were normal and symmetrical at the radial arteries. Reflexes were normal and symmetrical at the biceps, triceps, and brachioradialus tendons. Finger movements were markedly slow. She was unable to fully extend all of her fingers (digits). Flexion deformities at the PIPs existed, especially at the right third and fourth PIP joints, as well as the left third PIP joint. Sensory examination of the digits was grossly intact to light touch, pressure, as well as to pin prick, but with complaints of decreased sensation on the right side. Two point discrimination testing was diminished on the right, but somewhat inconsistent varying between 5–10 millimeters two point perception, especially decreased at the right thumb and index finger of the right hand. Capillary refill was brisk in all digits. No gross bony deformities were present at the wrists or hands. Upper extremity strength was generally decreased at the elbows, wrists, and forearms. This was more so on the right, but was also associated with give way weakness.

Hand strength grip testing was evaluated using a Jamar dynamometer. In the number 3 position while rapidly alternating strength testing between the right and left hands through a total of at least five cycles, the right hand strength varied between 10–19 pounds per square inch and the left hand grip strength varied between 12–34 pounds per square inch. Grip strength testing using the Jamar dynamometer throughout all positions did not yield the normally expected bell-shaped curve for either hand with the right hand strength varying between 9 and 14 pounds per square inch and left hand strength varying between 8 and 18 pounds per square inch. The results of grip strength testing using the Jamar dynamometer were not consistent with good examinee effort. It should be noted that according to the AMA's *Guides to the Evaluation of Permanent Impairment, Fourth Edition*, that the average grip strength for a 50–59 year old female should be approximately 49 pounds per square inch in the dominant hand and 40 pounds per square inch in the non-dominant hand. It is also noted that tests that are repeated at intervals are considered to be more reliable if there is less than 20% variation readings and that if there is more than a 20% variation, one may assume the patient is not exerting full effort. It should be noted that the variation in strength of Ms. XXXX's right hand was almost 100% when rapidly alternating the grip strength testing and more than 100% variation in her left hand. Thus, these results are not consistent with good examinee effort.

REVIEW OF MEDICAL RECORDS: One hundred and nine pages of medical records were reviewed.

1. Seventy-four pages of Ohio Bureau of Worker's Compensation C-141 forms were evaluated. These are wage loss statements for job search.
2. Seventeen pages of office notes, correspondence, as well as prescriptions from the ORTHOPEDIC PLACE were reviewed. These included at least 25 different office entries and were dated from October 30, 19XX through August 10, 2XXX. There were entries for every year. It should be noted that no mention of involvement concerning her hands was noted until July 8, 19XX when her pain was noted to extend from the base of her neck down into the arm and including the fingers and hands. It was also noted at that time that she had numbness and tingling in the hand. It was at this point in time that Dr. D desired obtaining electrodiagnostic studies of the right upper extremity and in his words, "To evaluate possible cervical radiculitis."
3. Nine pages of Ohio Bureau of Worker's Compensation forms were reviewed. These included C-84's, C-94A's, C-86's, C-9's, all signed by MS. XXXX or Dr. D. These forms dated between January 11, 19XX and August 15, 2XXX. The final work capacity form signed by Dr. D. Specifically the C-86 dated March 26, 19XX requested payments for loss wage benefits and requested additional allowances for major depressive disorder and generalized anxiety disorder as well as for authorization for outpatient psychotherapy treatment. The C-9 dated August 15, 2XXX requested allowance for carpal tunnel syndrome of the right upper extremity.

4. The job description and physical requirements of the position held by MS. XXXX at THE COMPANY completed by MS. XXXX from I M GROSS ATTORNEYS, LPA, dated January 21, 19XX was reviewed.
5. A psychological evaluation report dated January 11, 19XX completed by J M PING Conclusions was reviewed. Impressions were that MS. XXXX suffered from a major depressive disorder and general anxiety disorder which, based on his opinion, were disorders developed as a result of the injury of June 7, 19XX, and that MS. XXXX would require ongoing treatment and evaluation.
6. Correspondence from RISK E EVALUATORS' C. M. WORK, dated April 3, 2XXX, noting that the employer will approve the EMG and nerve conduction study for diagnostic purposes only.
7. Electrodiagnostic studies performed by Dr. H. dated May 26, 2XXX on the right upper extremity indicated that there was electrophysiologic evidence of moderate right carpal tunnel syndrome. These studies demonstrated no electrophysiologic evidence of cervical radiculopathy, brachioplexopathy, other entrapment neuropathy, polyneuropathy, or myopathy involving the right arm.

Diagnosis

1. Right lateral epicondylitis, 19XX.
2. Status post right rotator cuff tear and subsequent repair, 19XX.
3. Diagnosed with right shoulder tendonitis, 19XX.
4. Tendonitis of the right flexor carpiradialis, 2XXX.
5. Diagnosis of right carpal tunnel syndrome, 2XXX.
6. Obesity.
7. Diagnosed with depression and anxiety, 19XX.
8. Inflammation bilaterally of the hands and wrists, unknown etiology.

SUMMARY: The following conclusions are based on the available medical records, the history as supplied by Ms. XXXX, and the physical examination that I performed on November 15, 2XXX. It should be noted that the only allowed condition of this claim, of which I am aware, is for a right lateral epicondylitis. This was after contacting MANAGED CARE ORGANIZATION and speaking with the CASE MANAGER.

It is apparent by the information available that Ms. XXXX has had ongoing right elbow and right shoulder problem since 19XX. The right rotator cuff tear and subsequent repair has left Ms. XXXX with ongoing persistent pain problems in her right shoulder. It was apparent by the available medical records that Ms. XXXX had no complaints consistent with upper extremity neurological involvement until such was documented in October 19XX, when it was suggested that she may have a cervical radiculopathy. This was the first documented evidence of any possible neurological problems affecting Ms. XXXX or her right upper extremity. This leaves a gap of more than two years, from the time of the injury to the development of her hand symptoms. While it is true that some conditions develop because of a pre-existing condition, the belief that carpal tunnel is work related is primarily based on the concept of overuse, where occupational behaviors including heavy manual labor, repetitive stress or other injury are thought to be the predisposing (or definitive) cause of the development of an entrapment neuropathy, such as carpal tunnel syndrome.

The Medical Disability Advisor, Third Edition, warns that the diagnosis of carpal tunnel is controversial. *The Medical Disability Advisor* adds that causes <u>may</u> include highly repetitive wrist motion or sustained posturing of the wrist in awkward positions, but that the actual cause of carpal tunnel syndrome is swelling and inflammation about the nerve which may be caused by fluid retention, which itself can be related to late stages of pregnancy, menopause, use of birth control pills, hypothyroidism, fracture of the wrist or chronic inflammatory conditions such as rheumatoid arthritis among others. Additionally, diabetes is thought to be an additional risk factor for development of carpal tunnel syndrome. Obesity is also often believed to be a risk factor for the development of the condition.

In July 1997, the National Institute for Occupational Safety and Health made an attempt to review the literature regarding carpal tunnel syndrome (and other conditions). In their publication, *Musculoskeletal Disorders and Workplace Factors, a Critical Review*, of all the articles available for carpal tunnel syndrome at that time, six articles met their criteria for evaluation. The conclusions among the different articles varied between that there was no difference between low and high risk exposures, that there was some degree of risk associated with repetitiveness, that risk was associated with age rather than activity, to no association between either repetition or posture being a cause or effect of carpal tunnel syndrome. The conclusion's of this review is that there is weak, but not absent, evidence found for an association between occupation and the disease. Also absent in the review was a dose/effect relationship between the development of carpal tunnel syndrome and work, yet the evidence regarding specific occupational risk factors, such as force, repetition or posture were not consistently present with regard to the development of carpal tunnel syndrome. The concept that carpal tunnel syndrome should be considered a work related condition, although commonly accepted, is not 100%, as in fact more than half of all cases of carpal tunnel syndrome diagnosed are not considered to be work related.

In addition to this, Ms. XXXX has not worked for four years. By her own admission, she has been doing markedly less activity over the past several years, especially the past one to two years, than she did previously. She's been having pain as her primary complaint in both hands and wrists, with the numbness and tingling affecting her right upper extremity in a more pronounced manner in the past six months. According to an article in the *Journal of the Southwest Orthopedic Association*, by Robert R. Slater, Jr., M.D., titled "Carpal Tunnel Syndrome: Concepts," he too notes that occupation or job related hand or wrist overuse as risk factors for developing carpal tunnel is highly controversial. Dr. Slater noted that the most common symptom is paresthesias in the distribution of the median nerve. Although pain can be present, the presence of pain without paresthesias is much less common than the presence of paresthesias without pain. This means, at least by the statements that Ms. XXXX made, that she was having pain and discomfort in her upper extremities for a year or better before developing the numbness in her right hand.

Thus, I have several significant qualms with the idea that the development of Ms. XXXX's carpal tunnel syndrome would be directly or causally related to a specific incident that occurred more than four years previously. The June 7, 19XX work incident affected her right elbow and (apparently) also her right shoulder. She has multiple risk factors for the development of carpal tunnel syndrome including obesity, as well as an ongoing inflammatory process affecting her hands and wrists, which has not been evaluated to date or diagnosed. She also has a history of marked polyuria and nocturia, which although she stated that she does drink a lot of fluids, may be a sign of her having diabetes. She also has not been evaluated for the presence or absence of thyroid disease. Additionally, Ms. XXXX had no complaints of hand or wrist pain or paresthesias (numbness and tingling) for more than two years after the work related incident affected a distinctly separate anatomic area, her right elbow (and possibly also her right shoulder). **Therefore, it is my medical opinion that within a reasonable degree of certainty there has been shown no direct and causal relationship between the specific work related incident in 19XX and resultant injuries to her right elbow (and shoulder) and the development of carpal tunnel syndrome XX years later**.

I had informed Ms. XXXX that there would be no physician-patient relationship established during the course of this assessment, but I also told her that if I found anything of significance affecting her health, I would inform her of such information. Thus, as it is apparent that Ms. XXXX is suffering from an ongoing and markedly debilitating active inflammatory process affecting her wrists and hands, she was strongly advised to follow up with a rheumatologist at her earliest convenience.

I hope the above information has been helpful. If any additional information does become available, its review may or may not alter my conclusions contained within this report. If you have further questions related to this report, please feel free to contact me at your convenience.

Respectfully submitted,

Grumpy Oldie, M.D., FAADEP
Certified Independent Medical Examiner, ABIME

After Example - Using Color, Alternate Formatting, and Diagrams

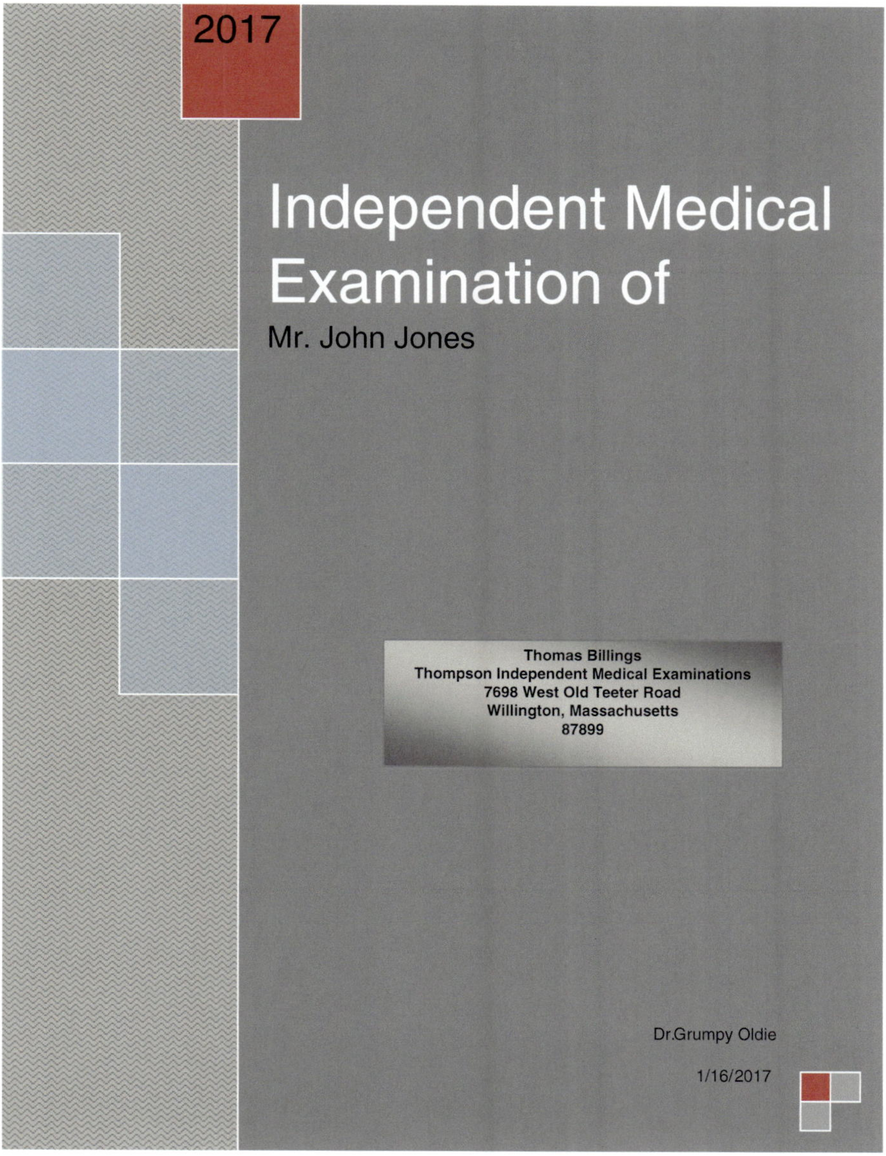

2017

Independent Medical Examination of

Mr. John Jones

Thomas Billings
Thompson Independent Medical Examinations
7698 West Old Teeter Road
Willington, Massachusetts
87899

Dr.Grumpy Oldie

1/16/2017

Report Table of Contents

Melbourne Orthopaedic Group

Robert C. Bantly MD
4998 South Winding Way
Suite 122
Melbourne, SC 89132
800-555-1212
rbently@melbooune.com

Date:

Managed Care Organization
Attn: Case Manager
Address
City, State Zip Code

Claimant:	Ms. XXXX
BWC Number:	
Date of Injury:	
Social Security Number:	
Employer:	THE COMPANY
Allowed Conditions:	Right Lateral Epicondylitis

Dear Case Manager:

At your request, I performed an independent medical examination on Ms. XXXX on November 15, 2XXX. It was explained to Ms. XXXX that the purpose of this examination was for evaluation purposes only and that no treatment would be undertaken. It was further explained to her that the client requesting and paying for the assessment would receive a report. Lastly, it was explained to Ms. XXXX that no medical relationship would be formed; thus no physician-patient relationship would be established during the course of this assessment.

A request is being made for an additional allowance of right carpal tunnel syndrome

CHIEF COMPLAINT: Hand pain and numbness.

HISTORY OF PRESENT ILLNESS: The following narrative was told to the examiner by Ms. XXXX and was dictated in her presence.

Ms. XXXX denied having an prior history of neck, upper back, shoulder, or upper extremity problems before 19XX. MS. XXXX worked intermittently for THE COMPANY since approximately 19XX. In 19XX she was rehired and worked at THE COMPANY continuously until 19XX.

THE COMPANY is now known as THE COMPANY. MS. XXXX worked as an equipment technician, where she ran a bender and/or saws. She stated that the bender machine did not run properly. She said when operating the bender, she would slide parts for framing windows. In the spring of 19XX the machine jerked and caused her to jerk her right arm.

She stated that she quickly had right lateral elbow swelling and pain, but that her entire arm also hurt. She was initially diagnosed as having tennis elbow. X-rays were performed. She was told to use a forearm or (tennis elbow) band. She had injections over a period of several visits.

At this point in time she was seeing her family doctor, but continued to work, usually seven days a week.

Ms. XXXX indicated that her elbow and arm continued to bother her, especially her shoulder. She complained of having shoulder pain at night, which would wake her. She stated that placing her shoulder and arm in a sling type position seemed to help decrease the discomfort. Once every other week, the pain in her right shoulder would become excruciating, at which time the pain would radiate into the right arm to the elbow. Using ice seemed to help, sometimes. The pain in the shoulder was so severe at times that she was unable to go to work.

One morning sometime in mid to late October 19XX, she could not use her shoulder because of severe pain and swelling. She thought that the last day she worked was October 13, 19XX. She followed up with Dr. K at her family physician's office, who referred her to an orthopedic surgeon, Dr. D. An arthrogram was subsequently performed and a tear in the right rotator cuff was found. She had surgery to repair the right rotator cuff in December 19XX (surgery had been delayed secondary to problems with her asthma and chronic bronchitis).

Ms. XXXX stated that she has had significant pain since before and after having surgery to her right shoulder. She stated the pain has not improved since surgery, but does wax and wane in severity. She attended six weeks of physical therapy at HHHH HOSPITAL and then eight additional weeks performing work hardening at CCCC CENTER. She underwent several nerve blocks, which relieved the pain only briefly. She also spent six weeks in the pain program at THE CENTER in Columbus, Ohio. She finished that program in September 19XX. She stated that the program did not help relieve her pain.

She has pain when lying on her shoulder, at night the pain wakes her up. She has severe pain approximately once a month. She had no improvement in shoulder movement after surgery. The severity of the shoulder pain varies significantly. She can be moderately pain free at rest. Using ice does help. Reaching forward is less bothersome than reaching laterally. Reaching behind her is especially bothersome.

She occasionally gets neck and right upper back pain and spasms. Pain worsens with lifting, such that she can no longer lift a one gallon jug of milk.

She has difficulty getting groceries out of her car. She has markedly decreased activities of daily living such as house cleaning, because of the shoulder pain and right upper extremity weakness.

She now has to get help performing her normal housekeeping chores. She had decreased sleep secondary to her shoulder problem, but it has worsened because of her recent hand difficulties.

Currently on Social Security Disability

She stated that she has been on Social Security Disability since 19XX. She is unable to lift like she used to. She is also unable to perform repetitive activities using her shoulders. Her right shoulder strength is markedly decreased. She stated that her right elbow has not been treated or evaluated since 19XX. The right elbow pain is not as severe as it was initially after the accident. The right elbow can be pain free for several days in a row.

The right elbow can be exacerbated with lifting type activities and can be painful for several days in a row.

She believes her right elbow has some swelling in it on a fairly persistent basis. She wears a forearm band which does seem to help when she has to lift.

She has had some right hand or other upper extremity difficulties for the past 9–12 months. Her right hand, including all digits and the thumb, can go numb. This can occur during the day, but especially happens at night. It can wake her several times a night and the numbness can be present when she wakes up in the morning.

She also noted that she has recurrent right hand swelling. She noted that this numbness can last for a while. She said because of her right upper extremity difficulties she has been using her left hand more (especially since the shoulder injury). She denied having any left handed numbness, but she has had pain at the ulnar side of the left wrist and hand for several months.

Diagnosis of Carpal Tunnel Syndrome ~ Surgery Recommended

Dr. D has been evaluating her for her upper extremity difficulties and had wanted to do electrodiagnostic testing of the right upper extremity. This was not completed until May 2XXX, when testing by Dr. H demonstrated right carpal tunnel syndrome. Dr. D advised her to undergo carpal tunnel release, but she is not certain if she wants this performed. She has been dropping objects with both hands. She has recurrent hand swelling, the right usually worse than the left. The left has been bothering her more recently. She uses a wrist splint on the right side at night which helps decrease her symptoms. She also uses a left wrist band, which helps support her left wrist.

She recently lifted a jewelry box, maybe 5 pounds in weight, with her left hand. She ended up dropping the box. It twisted her left wrist, which increased her left wrist pain. She specifically denied ever having any injuries to her upper extremities since 1996.

As part of this claim, she stated that she has been seen for both depression and anxiety. She has been treated by a psychologist for this condition.

She denied having any testing for thyroid, arthritis, or diabetes. She stated that she has had a 20–30 pound weight loss over the past year. She complained of having decreased weight, decreased sleep, decreased appetite, but denied having any fevers.

She stated that she has nocturia, which has increased recently, although she indicated that she has also increased her fluid intake recently.

During the discussion with Ms. XXXX regarding the development of her symptoms, she persistently reiterated that she had no problems with her hands until after she had injured her right upper extremity. She noted that she has had a gradual onset of bilateral hand and wrist symptoms over the past several years.

No New Incident Reported During Time Frame of Interest

She specifically denied any new incident or injury to her upper extremities during this time frame. Over the past year, she has been less able to extend her fingers. This has worsened to the point where she is no longer able to fully extend certain fingers of both hands. Her hands are very stiff in the morning. This can last easily for half an hour or longer. She stated that some mornings she has to pry her fingers open. She complained of having ongoing finger pain and stiffness, as well as wrist pain and stiffness.

She has recurrent swelling in her distal upper extremities, primarily involving the hands and fingers. She reiterated that her right hand is worse than her left, but that the left has very similar if not identical symptoms to the right, except for the lack of tingling and numbness.

Past Medical History

Ms. XXXX has undergone the following surgeries:

1. surgical repair of her right earlobe,
2. 19XX; hysterectomy, bilateral salpingo-oophorectomy,
3. and appendectomy, 19XX;
4. low back surgery (L3-4, L4-5) with residual left leg symptoms from nerve damage, 19XX;

   Right rotator cuff repair, 19XX.

Ms. XXXX Has the Following Medical Conditions

1. She has been hospitalized for hemoptysis,
2. 19XX and for hypertension, 19XX.
3. Other past medical problems have included a history of sinus and allergy problems since 19XX;
4. diagnosis of irritable bowel syndrome in 19XX;
5. history of recurrent bladder infections;
6. a history of gastric ulcers times two, 19XX or 19XX, also associated with gastritis and accompanying esophageal stricture, status post dilation.
7. She also was diagnosed with hypertension,
8. 19XX; diagnosed with asthma, 19XX;
9. diagnosed with coronary artery disease with a 50% posterior coronary block,
10. 19XX; and diagnosed with depression and anxiety, 19XX.
11. Past musculoskeletal problems include a removal of a ganglionic cyst from her right hand in the 19XXs,
12. the low back injury with resultant surgery in 19XX,
13. diagnosis of left knee bursitis requiring drainage in 19XX,

14. the diagnosis of tennis elbow in 19XX,
15. the right rotator cuff tear and rotator cuff repair in 19XX,
16. diagnosis of right shoulder tendonitis,
17. 19XX; diagnosis of right forearm tendonitis,
18. 2XXX and diagnosis of carpal tunnel syndrome,
19. 2XXX. Medications include Prilosec, Ultram, Soma compound, Elavil, Allegra, Tenormin, Albuterol, Singulair, Flovent, Seravent, Estratab, and an aspirin a day.
20. She denied having any allergies to medications.

FAMILY HISTORY: There is a family history of high blood pressure, heart attack, stroke, bleeding problems, ulcers, obesity, birth defects, diabetes, cerebral palsy, asbestosis and cancer. Her father is deceased at the age of __ years from asbestos disease and cancer. Her mother is alive and well at the age of __ years. She has ____ brothers, ages ______ who are all alive and well, except that the oldest and youngest both have diabetes. She has ____ living children, ages_______. A sixth child was born with cerebral palsy and died in 19XX. She is currently divorced from her only marriage.

SOCIAL HISTORY: She has not smoked in 5–6 years, but does have a 15–20 pack year smoking history. She does not consume alcohol and denied recreational drug use. She does enjoy reading, primarily the bible. She occasionally plays card games or checkers with her grandchildren. She denied performing any repetitive hand activities as far as hobbies. She denied performing any regular exercise, although she does try to walk once a week. She has no pets at home. She wears glasses.

OCCUPATIONAL HISTORY: Ms. XXXX worked at ANOTHER COMPANY in SOMEPLACE, Ohio from 19XX – 19XX doing spot welding on an automatic sealer. After that she worked at ANOTHER PLACE cleaning offices from 19XX – 19XX. She also worked at A NURSING HOME as a nursing assistant from 19XX – 19XX.

She worked continuously at THE COMPANY (formerly THE COMPANY) from 19XX – 19XX, and also worked there previously on an intermittent basis and during lay-offs she worked at nursing homes.

She has had past occupational exposures to grinding dust, metal dust, other dust, engine exhaust, smoke, other fumes mists or vapors, ammonia, welding fumes, acids and/or caustics, oils, metal coolants, viruses, noise, cold, heavy lifting, change in shift work, repetitive mechanical work and poor lighting.

REVIEW OF SYSTEMS: She is a gravida X, para X, with X living children. She has a history of bleeding problems. There is a history of hemophilia in the family. She has trouble sleeping. She has intermittently blurry vision. She has persistent ringing in her ears since 19XX. She has a history of sinus problems.

She has a history of cough, some shortness of breath at rest, recurrent wheezing and congestion. She has coughed up blood in the past, including while at work in 19XX-19XX. She has a history of chest pain, but this has been less since resuming female replacement hormones. She also has a history of heart flutter and a history of high blood pressure. She complains of having a change of appetite and of having heart burn.

She does get up a lot at night to urinate. She has complaints of anxiety, depression, confusion, and memory problems. She has a history of pain, swelling, or stiffness in her joints, arthritis, pain or numbness in her extremities, of having muscle cramps, of having low back pain or stiffness, of having neck pain or stiffness, of having swelling in her ankles, and of having some joint deformities and decreased function.

PAIN ASSESSMENT: On the Borg's pain scale, she rated her current pain as a 5. On the Borg's pain scale, 0 is no pain at all and 10 is a very very strong pain. She indicated that over the past 30 days her best level of pain was a level 5 and at it's worst it was a level 8. She stated that she is more limited by her hand movements than the pain. With further questioning, she noted that she did not get pain in the tip of her tailbone, that her whole leg does not become painful, nor does it go numb, nor does it give away.

She did indicate that she has not had any spells with very little pain during the past year. These answers were not the same as those when she initially answered the questionnaire. On the Visual Analogue Pain Scale, she marked near the 50% mark, which correlates with her responses on the Borg's Analogue Pain Scale. Her responses on the McGill Pain Questionnaire totaled 33, which demonstrates a tendency to abnormal psychodynamics. Her responses on the Ransford Pain Drawing are consistent with the stated complaints. Ms. XXXX's responses using the pain assessment tools do not indicate significant pain symptom magnification, but are not entirely normal.

Physical Examination

General

This was a well-developed, well-nourished right hand dominant over weight 54 year old black female with short black hair and glasses. Her vital signs were all normal except for mildly elevated blood pressure at 152/96. Her height was 5′ 6 ½″ tall. Her weight was 217 pounds. Although she was pleasant and cooperative throughout the interview process and during the examination, her responses seemed somewhat delayed. Her affect appeared flat. In general, she appeared to be somewhat depressed.

Gait and Motion

She ambulated somewhat slowly with a wide based gait and a slight limp. Neck range of motion was mildly decreased, especially left lateral bending.

No guarding was observed during active neck range of motion. There was no pain elicited with gentle cervical compression. No masses were palpated in the neck.

Spinal Examination

There was posterior cervical paraspinal muscle tenderness palpated especially at both occiputs, as well as point tenderness of the central right cervical paraspinal muscles. There was tenderness to palpation of the right rhomboid, right trapezius, and right infraspinatus muscles. There was no tenderness to palpation of the cervical or thoracic spine. Back range of motion was fair with some decreased anterior flexion and lateral bending. No scapular winging was appreciated. A well healed lower mid-line surgical back scar was visualized.

Multiple Tender Points Reported

Multiple tender points were palpated including over the left greater trochanter, left buttock, both trapezius muscles, at the occiput bilaterally, both rhomboids, at the right anterior chest, right deltoid, and right dorsal forearm. A well-healed surgical scar was visualized over the anterior portion of the right shoulder.

Active Shoulder Range of Motion: revealed the following:

(a) Right shoulder abduction was 80°
(b) Left shoulder abduction was 120° (normal being 170°+).
(c) Right shoulder adduction was 10°
(d) Left shoulder adduction was 30° (normal being 50°).
(e) Right shoulder flexion was 90°
(f) Left shoulder flexion was 135° (normal being 180°)
(g) At 90° of abduction (somewhat less on the right),
(h) Left external and internal rotation reached 45°, (normal internal rotation being 80° or greater,
(i) External rotation being 60° or greater).
(j) Right internal shoulder rotation at approximately 80° of shoulder abduction, reached 35° with the above normals previously being described.
(k) No right shoulder external rotation was elicited.
(l) No shoulder laxity was elicited.
(m) There was tenderness to palpation of the right anterior chest, throughout the right glenohumeral joint, the right acromioclavicular joint and right deltoid.

The anterior chest and deltoid tenderness was limited to point tenderness. There was no right arm or clavicle tenderness to palpation. No obvious swelling, deformity, or atrophy was appreciated, except at the hands. There was marked decreased strength of the right shoulder and was associated with give way weakness.

A well healed scar was visualized on the left dorsal radial wrist.

Upper Extremity Examination

There was tenderness to palpation of the left wrist, at the anatomic stuff box, and of the left hand, especially at the metacarpal phalangeal joints, and over the second through fifth proximal interphalangeal (PIP) finger joints.

This tenderness was slightly less over the third PIP. There was also slight discomfort to palpation at the left distal interphalangeal finger joints. There was some slight swelling throughout the hands and wrists primarily over the metacarpal phalangeal joints and fingers. No thenar atrophy was appreciated.

There was also tenderness to palpation over the right wrist, right anatomic stuff box, and over the right metacarpal phalangeal finger joints and second and third proximal interphalangeal finger joints. The right hand swelling was similar to that of the left. She complained of mildly decreased sensation throughout the fingers and thumb of the right hand, especially over the thumb, third and second digits. She had markedly decreased grip strength bilaterally. She also had markedly decreased opposition of her thumb with the fourth and fifth fingers, especially on the right.

No crepitus was appreciated of either upper extremity. There was decreased supination bilaterally and decreased wrist flexion and extension, especially on the left. Finklestein's maneuver elicited no symptoms bilaterally. Elbow flexion appeared to be mildly decreased but was symmetrical, with decreased elbow extension, the right reaching 160° while the left reaching 170° (normal being 180°). There was tenderness to palpation of the right lateral epicondyle and into the adjacent dorsal forearm, but not at the olecranon or antecubital fossa. Pulses were normal and symmetrical at the radial arteries.

Tendon Reflexes

Reflexes were normal and symmetrical at the biceps, triceps, and brachioradialus tendons.

Finger movements were markedly slow. She was unable to fully extend all of her fingers (digits). Flexion deformities at the PIPs existed, especially at the right third and fourth PIP joints, as well as the left third PIP joint. Sensory examination of the digits was grossly intact to light touch, pressure, as well as to pin prick, but with complaints of decreased sensation on the right side.

Sensation and Strength

Two point discrimination testing was diminished on the right, but somewhat inconsistent varying between 5–10 millimeters two point perception, especially decreased at the right thumb and index finger of the right hand. Capillary refill was brisk in all digits. No gross bony deformities were present at the wrists or hands. Upper extremity strength was generally decreased at the elbows, wrists, and forearms. This was more so on the right, but was also associated with give way weakness.

Hand strength grip testing was evaluated using a Jamar dynamometer. In the number 3 position while rapidly alternating strength testing between the right and left hands through a total of at least five cycles, the right hand strength varied between 10–19 pounds per square inch and the left hand grip strength varied between 12–34 pounds per square inch. Grip strength testing using the Jamar dynamometer throughout all positions did not yield the normally expected bell-shaped curve for either hand with the right hand strength varying between 9 and 14 pounds per square inch and left hand strength varying between 8 and 18 pounds per square inch.

The results of grip strength testing using the Jamar dynamometer were not consistent with good examinee effort.

AMA Guides Grip Strength Data

It should be noted that according to the AMA's *Guides to the Evaluation of Permanent Impairment, Fourth Edition*, that the average grip strength for a 50–59 year old female should be approximately 49 pounds per square inch in the dominant hand and 40 pounds per square inch in the non-dominant hand. It is also noted that tests that are repeated at intervals are considered to be more reliable if there is less than 20% variation readings and that if there is more than a 20% variation, one may assume the patient is not exerting full effort. It should be noted that the variation in strength of Ms. XXXX's right hand was almost 100% when rapidly alternating the grip strength testing and more than 100% variation in her left hand. Thus, these results are not consistent with good examinee effort.

Review of Medical Records

One hundred and nine pages of medical records were reviewed.

1. Seventy-four pages of Ohio Bureau of Worker's Compensation C-141 forms were evaluated. These are wage loss statements for job search.
2. Seventeen pages of office notes, correspondence, as well as prescriptions from the ORTHOPEDIC PLACE were reviewed. These included at least 25 different office entries and were dated from October 30, 19XX through August 10, 2XXX. There were entries for every year. It should be noted that no mention of involvement concerning her hands was noted until July 8, 19XX when her pain was noted to extend from the base of her neck down into the arm and including the fingers and hands. It was also noted at that time that she had numbness and tingling in the hand. It was at this point in time that Dr. D desired obtaining electrodiagnostic studies of the right upper extremity and in his words, "To evaluate possible cervical radiculitis."
3. Nine pages of Ohio Bureau of Worker's Compensation forms were reviewed. These included C-84's, C-94A's, C-86's, C-9's, all signed by MS. XXXX or Dr. D. These forms dated between January 11, 19XX and August 15, 2XXX. The final work capacity form signed by Dr. D. Specifically the C-86 dated March 26, 19XX requested payments for loss wage benefits and requested additional allowances for major depressive disorder and generalized anxiety disorder as well as for authorization for outpatient psychotherapy treatment. The C-9 dated August 15, 2XXX requested allowance for carpal tunnel syndrome of the right upper extremity.
4. The job description and physical requirements of the position held by MS. XXXX at THE COMPANY completed by MS. XXXX from I M GROSS ATTORNEYS, LPA, dated January 21, 19XX was reviewed.
5. A psychological evaluation report dated January 11, 19XX completed by J M PING Conclusions was reviewed.
   Impressions were that MS. XXXX suffered from a major depressive disorder and general anxiety disorder which, based on his opinion, were disorders developed as a result of the injury of June 7, 19XX, and that MS. XXXX would require ongoing treatment and evaluation.
6. Correspondence from RISK E EVALUATORS' C. M. WORK, dated April 3, 2XXX, noting that the employer will approve the EMG and nerve conduction study for diagnostic purposes only.

7. Electrodiagnostic studies performed by Dr. H. dated May 26, 2XXX on the right upper extremity indicated that there was electrophysiologic evidence of moderate right carpal tunnel syndrome.
   These studies demonstrated no electrophysiologic evidence of cervical radiculopathy, brachioplexopathy, other entrapment neuropathy, polyneuropathy, or myopathy involving the right arm.

Diagnosis

1. Right lateral epicondylitis, 19XX.
2. Status post right rotator cuff tear and subsequent repair, 19XX.
3. Diagnosed with right shoulder tendonitis, 19XX.
4. Tendonitis of the right flexor carpiradialis, 2XXX.
5. Diagnosis of right carpal tunnel syndrome, 2XXX.
6. Obesity.
7. Diagnosed with depression and anxiety, 19XX.
8. Inflammation bilaterally of the hands and wrists, unknown etiology.

Summary

The following conclusions are based on the available medical records, the history as supplied by Ms. XXXX, and the physical examination that I performed on November 15, 2XXX. It should be noted that the only allowed condition of this claim, of which I am aware, is for a right lateral epicondylitis. This was after contacting MANAGED CARE ORGANIZATION and speaking with the CASE MANAGER.

It is apparent by the information available that Ms. XXXX has had ongoing right elbow and right shoulder problem since 19XX. The right rotator cuff tear and subsequent repair has left Ms. XXXX with ongoing persistent pain problems in her right shoulder.

It was apparent by the available medical records that Ms. XXXX had no complaints consistent with upper extremity neurological involvement until such was documented in October 19XX, when it was suggested that she may have a cervical radiculopathy.

This was the first documented evidence of any possible neurological problems affecting Ms. XXXX or her right upper extremity. This leaves a gap of more than two years, from the time of the injury to the development of her hand symptoms. While it is true that some conditions develop because of a pre-existing condition, the belief that carpal tunnel is work related is primarily based on the concept of overuse, where occupational behaviors including heavy manual labor, repetitive stress or other injury are thought to be the predisposing (or definitive) cause of the development of an entrapment neuropathy, such as carpal tunnel syndrome.

The Medical Disability Advisor, Third Edition, warns that the diagnosis of carpal tunnel is controversial. *The Medical Disability Advisor* adds that causes may include highly repetitive wrist motion or sustained posturing of the wrist in awkward positions, but that the actual cause of carpal tunnel syndrome is swelling and inflammation about the nerve which may be caused by fluid retention, which itself can be related to late stages of pregnancy, menopause, use of birth control pills, hypothyroidism, fracture of the wrist or chronic inflammatory conditions such as rheumatoid arthritis among others. Additionally, diabetes is thought to be an additional risk factor for development of carpal tunnel syndrome. Obesity is also often believed to be a risk factor for the development of the condition.

In July 1997, the National Institute for Occupational Safety and Health made an attempt to review the literature regarding carpal tunnel syndrome (and other conditions). In their publication, *Musculoskeletal Disorders and Workplace Factors, a Critical Review*, of all the articles available for carpal tunnel syndrome at that time, six articles met their criteria for evaluation.

The conclusions among the different articles varied between that there was no difference between low and high risk exposures, that there was some degree of risk associated with repetitiveness, that risk was associated with age rather than activity, to no association between either repetition or posture being a cause or effect of carpal tunnel syndrome. The conclusion's of this review is that there is weak, but not absent, evidence found for an association between occupation and the disease.

Also absent in the review was a dose /effect relationship between the development of carpal tunnel syndrome and work, yet the evidence regarding specific occupational risk factors, such as force, repetition or posture were not consistently present with regard to the development of carpal tunnel syndrome. The concept that carpal tunnel syndrome should be considered a work related condition, although commonly accepted, is not 100%, as in fact more than half of all cases of carpal tunnel syndrome diagnosed are not considered to be work related.

In addition to this, Ms. XXXX has not worked for four years. By her own admission, she has been doing markedly less activity over the past several years, especially the past one to two years, than she did previously.

She's been having pain as her primary complaint in both hands and wrists, with the numbness and tingling affecting her right upper extremity in a more pronounced manner in the past six months. According to an article in the *Journal of the Southwest Orthopedic Association*, by Robert R. Slater, Jr., M.D., titled "Carpal Tunnel Syndrome: Concepts," he too notes that occupation or job related hand or wrist overuse as risk factors for developing carpal tunnel is highly controversial.

Dr. Slater noted that the most common symptom is paresthesias in the distribution of the median nerve. Although pain can be present, the presence of pain without paresthesias is much less common than the presence of parasthesias without pain. This means, at least by the statements that Ms. XXXX made, that she was having pain and discomfort in her upper extremities for a year or better before developing the numbness in her right hand.

Thus, I have several significant qualms with the idea that the development of Ms. XXXX's carpal tunnel syndrome would be directly or causally related to a specific incident that occurred more than four years previously. The June 7, 19XX work incident affected her right elbow and (apparently) also her right shoulder.

She has multiple risk factors for the development of carpal tunnel syndrome including obesity, as well as an ongoing inflammatory process affecting her hands and wrists, which has not been evaluated to date or diagnosed. She also has a history of marked polyuria and nocturia, which although she stated that she does drink a lot of fluids, may be a sign of her having diabetes. She also has not been evaluated for the presence or absence of thyroid disease. Additionally, Ms. XXXX had no complaints of hand or wrist pain or paresthesias (numbness and tingling) for more than two years after the work related incident affected a distinctly separate anatomic area, her right elbow (and possibly also her right shoulder).

Medical Analysis Conclusion

Therefore, it is my medical opinion that within a reasonable degree of certainty there has been shown no direct and causal relationship between the specific work related incident in 19XX and resultant injuries to her right elbow (and shoulder) and the development of carpal tunnel syndrome XX years later.

I had informed Ms. XXXX that there would be no physician-patient relationship established during the course of this assessment, but I also told her that if I found anything of significance affecting her health, I would inform her of such information. Thus, as it is apparent that Ms. XXXX is suffering from an ongoing and markedly debilitating active inflammatory process affecting her wrists and hands, she was strongly advised to follow up with a rheumatologist at her earliest convenience.

I hope the above information has been helpful. If any additional information does become available, its review may or may not alter my conclusions contained within this report. If you have further questions related to this report, please feel free to contact me at your convenience.

Respectfully submitted,

Grumpy Oldie, M.D., FAADEP

Certified Independent Medical Examiner, ABIME

Report Word Index

The Medical Disability Advisor

Epicondylitis, Medial and Lateral

Duration | Trends | Rehabilitation | Codes | UMK | Costs   Go ... | Bookmark | Print

Related Terms: Golfer's Elbow, Tennis Elbow

- **Definition**

Epicondylitis occurs when tendons in the elbow develop inflammation, and ultimately microscopic tears and degeneration.

Many of the muscles and tendons responsible for wrist and finger movements attach in the elbow region to the upper arm bone (humerus). The areas of attachment are the bony prominences just above the elbow joint (epicondyles). The tendons develop inflammation and sometimes microscopic tears. This process is known as epicondylitis. It can occur on either on the outside (lateral) or inside (medial) face of the elbow. It is more commonly known as "tennis elbow" when on the lateral side and "golfer's elbow" when on the medial side. Medial epicondylitis accounts for only about 10% to 20% of all epicondylitis (Young).

Although the cause is unknown, epicondylitis may be a result of overuse or overexertion of the forearm and wrist muscles. Up to half of all tennis players may experience epicondylitis (Disabella).

Risk: Risk increases with occupations and sports that require a repetitive or stressful movement of the forearm. Epicondylitis typically afflicts individuals between the ages of 20 and 40. Although men are twice as likely to develop medial epicondylitis as women, lateral epicondylitis affects men and women equally (Mercier).

Incidence and Prevalence: Lateral is 5 times more common than medial epicondylitis (Mercier). The exact incidence is difficult to determine, although it is estimated that lateral epicondylitis occurs in about 6 per 1,000 industrial workers (Disabella).

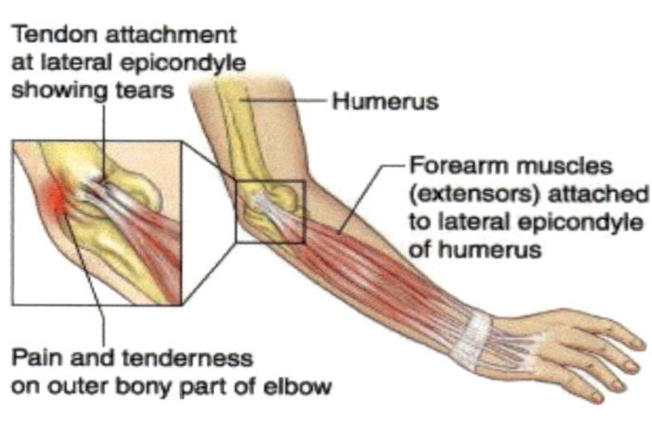

- **Diagnosis**

  History: Individuals commonly report elbow pain with forceful gripping, swelling, and decreased ability to use the wrist of one arm (frequently the dominant arm). The symptoms may appear suddenly, but more often the onset is gradual and progressive. Pain is localized to the elbow region initially, but may progress to involve the muscle mass of the forearm. Individuals may relate a change in activity or increase in size and weight of tools used immediately preceding the pain. Most cases, however, occur without an obvious cause. History of neck and shoulder injuries should be noted.

  Physical exam: On physical examination, pain may be localized over either epicondyle and may increase with resisted wrist motion. Bending the wrist forward against resistance (flexion) causes pain for individuals with medial epicondylitis and bending the wrist backward against resistance (extension) causes pain for those with lateral epicondylitis. Passive stretch of the involved muscle/tendon units also causes pain. As the condition becomes more chronic, pain and weakness may involve the forearm as well, especially with resisted wrist and finger motion.

  Tests: An injection test, in which a local anesthetic is injected into the most tender point of the elbow, may suggest the diagnosis if the elbow pain is relieved by the injection. When the diagnosis is in doubt or if an individual fails to respond to treatment, x-rays are done to rule out bony abnormalities about the joint. MRI may show abnormal signals in the medial or lateral epicondyle but is usually unnecessary.

- **Treatment**

  Initial conservative treatment consists of rest from the precipitating or exacerbating activity, generally anti-inflammatory medication for pain and inflammation, and a band around the proximal forearm (forearm strap or counter-force brace). The forearm strap spreads the force of the muscle contraction over a greater area, and diminishes tensile stresses on the common extensor tendon (lateral epicondylitis) or common flexor tendon (medial epicondylitis). A wrist extension (cock-up) splint may be helpful in more severe cases. Ice often relieves pain after activity, with or without swelling. Massage may be beneficial. Stretching can be started immediately and strengthening exercises as the pain subsides.

  Local anesthetic-corticosteroid injection may be used in individuals who do not improve after a few weeks of treatment. The injection may not be fully effective for 5 to 7 days and can be repeated. Splints provide restriction of both the wrist and elbow and can be used in individuals not responding to other methods of treatment.

  Surgery is rarely necessary, but may be performed on individuals with pain lasting longer than 6 months despite appropriate nonoperative treatment. Surgery usually involves open release of the tendon's origin, excision of degenerated tendon and/or inflammatory tissue, and repair of any tendon gaps or tears. Any abnormalities in the elbow joint may be addressed concurrently.

- **Prognosis**

  Although recovery may be slow and tedious, most individuals have relief of all symptoms 1 year from onset. Conservative measures (i.e., nonsurgical) can relieve symptoms in more than 90% of the cases. Surgery relieves symptoms for more than 80% of individuals (Young), although some individuals experience pain during aggressive activities. Ulnar nerve involvement is associated with a poor prognosis. Recurrence of epicondylitis later in life is common.

- **Utilization Management Knowledgebase**
  ELB501 Epicondylitis, Medial
  ELB517 Epicondylitis, Lateral

- **Differential Diagnoses**
  Calcium deposits (calcification)
  Cervical radiculopathy
  Compartment syndrome
  Fracture
  Infection
  Inflammatory disease (rheumatoid arthritis, etc.)
  Intra-articular elbow pathology (osteoarthritis, osteochondritis dissecans)
  Irritation of the radial or ulnar nerve around the elbow (e.g., nerve entrapment)
  Ligament injuries
  Loose bodies
  Medial collateral ligament instability
  Pain traveling from another site (referred pain)
  Radial nerve compression
  Ulnar neuropathy

- **Specialists**
  Hand Surgeon
  Occupational Therapist
  Orthopedic (Orthopaedic) Surgeon
  Physiatrist
  Physical Therapist
  Rheumatologist
  Sports Medicine Internist

- **Rehabilitation**
  Note on research and authorship

The primary focus of rehabilitation for medial and lateral epicondylitis is to control pain and restore function. Modalities such as cold packs may be helpful in controlling painful symptoms. Loss of motion is usually not a problem with epicondylitis. However, individuals may avoid full range of motion as a result of excessive pain. During the initial period of acute symptomatology, advise individuals to avoid any movements that exacerbate pain. Occasionally, a resting splint may be recommended. Stretching and strengthening exercises of the wrist and extrinsic hand muscles may be beneficial and, when performed in conjunction with modalities, may provide relief. Home exercises should be taught as well as pain control measure (heat and cold).

There is some evidence to support the use of topical non-steroidal anti-inflammatory agents for epicondylitis (Green), and further evidence to support treatment with iontophoresis (Nirschl) or ultrasound (Smidt, "Effectiveness of Physiotherapy") for relief of symptoms. Local corticosteroid injections can provide short term relief (Hart). However, physical therapy may be more successful in the long term outcome of epicondylitis (Hart; Smidt, "Corticosteroid Injections").

It is advisable to consider work and leisure activities that may have contributed to the condition and attempt to reduce the risk factors associated with epicondylitis (Haahr). An ergonomic evaluation may be beneficial if work tasks are suspected as a cause (Lewis).

FREQUENCY OF REHABILITATION VISITS

Nonsurgical	
Specialist	Epicondylitis, Medial and Lateral
Physical or Occupational Therapist	Up to 8 visits within 4 weeks

The table above represents a range of the usual acceptable number of visits for uncomplicated cases. It provides a framework based on the duration of tissue healing time and standard clinical practice.

- **Comorbid Conditions**
  Arthritis
  Carpal tunnel syndrome
  Cervical spine disease
  Other injuries to the arm and shoulder.

- **Complications**
  Radial neuropathy occurs in less than a small percentage of the cases of lateral epicondylitis. Ulnar neuropathy (cubital tunnel syndrome) is some what more likely to occur in of the cases of medial epicondylitis. After local injections, there may be a 1 or 2 day increase in pain called postinjection flare.

- **Factors Influencing Duration**
  Duration of disability depends on job requirements (use of wrist, forearm), dominant versus nondominant arm work requirements, conservative versus surgical treatment, and compliance to rehabilitation program. Disability may be longer for individuals with job duties that require intensive use of both arms or repetitive actions.

- **Length of Disability**

Supportive treatment, medial and lateral epicondylitis

DURATION IN DAYS

Job Classification	Minimum	Optimum	Maximum
Sedentary	0	7	28
Light	1	10	28
Medium	7	21	56
Heavy	14	28	56
Very Heavy	14	28	56

• **Duration Trend from Reference Data**

DURATION TRENDS

ICD-9-CM: 726.31, 726.32

Cases	Mean	Min	Max	No Lost Time	Over 6 Months
1373	60	0	272	0.2%	5.8%

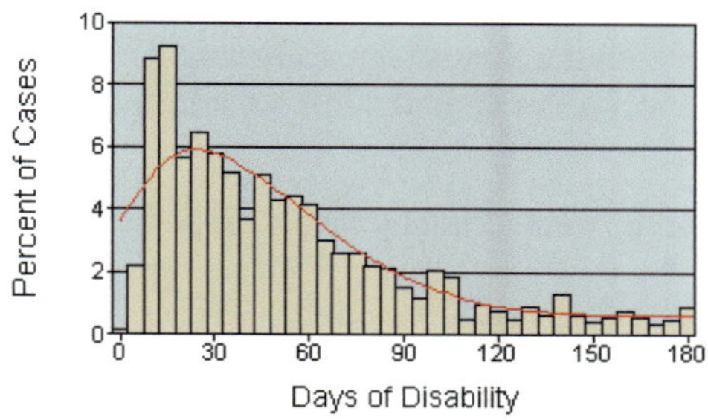

Percentile:	5th	25th	Median	75th	95th
Days:	7	20	42	78	182

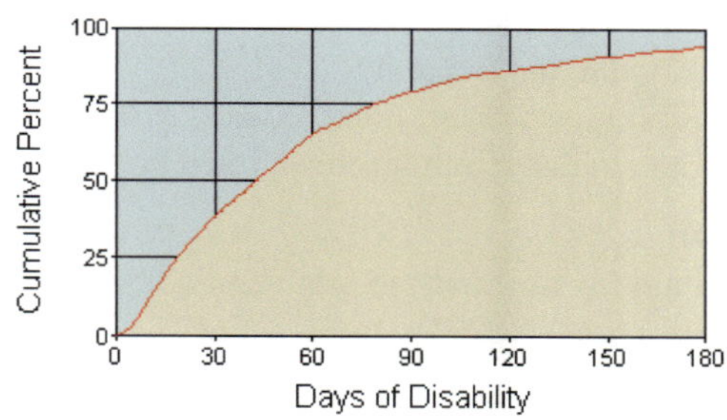

Differences may exist between the duration tables and the reference graphs. Duration tables provide expected recovery periods based on the type of work performed by the individual. The reference graphs reflect the actual experience of many individuals across the spectrum of physical conditions, in a variety of industries, and with varying levels of case management. Selected graphs combine multiple codes based on similar means and medians.

• **Return to Work (Restrictions / Accommodations)**

An ergonomic evaluation of the workplace may be necessary. The precipitating or exacerbating activity needs to be avoided until symptoms are relieved. Change in job duties, sharing or alternating tasks, and limiting time and frequency of repetitive activities are important accommodations. Use of vibrating tools such as impact wrenches or jackhammers should be minimized. Increasing or decreasing the size of tool grips so the wrist can be held in the "ideal" position is also helpful. Use of splints, straps, and casts affect dexterity and the individual may be temporarily unable to lift and carry heavy or bulky objects, operate equipment, or perform other tasks requiring the use of both hands. If the dominant arm was affected, the individual may be unable to write legibly, type well, or perform activities that require fine motor skills such as those in a laboratory or assembly line. Prescribed medications for pain and inflammation require evaluation of safety issues and drug policies.

- **Failure to Recover**

If an individual fails to recover within the maximum duration expectancy period, the reader may wish to reference the following questions to assist in better understanding the specifics of an individual's medical case.

Regarding diagnosis:

Does individual's occupation or hobby involve repetitive and/or stressful use of the forearm?

Does individual report elbow pain, swelling, and the inability to use the wrist and arm?

Has pain spread to the forearm?

Is the affected elbow on the dominant or nondominant side?

Does individual have a history of neck or shoulder injuries?

On physical examination, is the pain localized over either epicondyle?

Does pain increase with resisted wrist motion?

Is there weakness noted in the forearm?

Did individual have an injection test done? X-ray? MRI?

Have conditions with similar symptoms been ruled out?

Regarding treatment:

Has individual responded favorably to treatment consisting of rest from the aggravating activity, ice packs, NSAIDs, and a splint?

Has individual received a corticosteroid injection?

Was surgery necessary?

Regarding prognosis:

Is individual active in physical therapy? Does individual have a home exercise program?

Is individual's employer able to accommodate any necessary restrictions?

Has individual had an ergonomic evaluation of their work area?

Does individual have any conditions that may affect the ability to recover?

Does individual have any complications such as radial or ulnar neuropathy?

Did individual have a postinjection flare?

- **Medical Codes**

ICD-9-CM:	726.31, 726.32
ICD-10:	M77, M77.1

- **Cited References**

Disabella, Vincent N. "Lateral Epicondylitis." *eMedicine.com.* Eds. A. D. Perron, et al. 26 Oct. 2004.eMedicine.com, Inc. 8 Feb. 2005 <http://www.emedicine.com/sports/topic59.htm>.

Green, S., et al. "Non-Steroidal Anti-Inflammatory Drugs (NSAIDs) for Treating Lateral Elbow Pain in Adults." *Cochrane Database System Review* 2 (2002): CD003686. *National Center for Biotechnology Information.*National Library of Medicine. 17 Nov. 2004 <PMID: 12076503>.

Haahr, J. P., and J. H. Andersen. "Prognostic Factors in Lateral Epicondylitis: A Randomized Trial with One-Year Follow-Up in 266 New Cases Treated with minimal Occupational Intervention or the Usual Approach in General Practice." *Rheumatology* 42 10 (2003): 1216–1225. *National Center for Biotechnology Information.*National Library of Medicine. 17 Nov. 2004 <PMID: 12810936>.

Hart, L. E. "Corticosteroid Injections, Physiotherapy, or a Wait-and-See Policy for Lateral Epicondylitis?" *Clinical Journal of Sports Medicine* 12 6 (2002): 403–404. *National Center for Biotechnology Information.*National Library of Medicine. 17 Nov. 2004 <PMID: 12650155>.

Lewis, M., et al. "Effects of Manual Work on Recovery from Lateral Epicondylitis." *Scandinavian Journal of Work, Environment and Health* 28 2 (2002): 109–116. *National Center for Biotechnology Information.*National Library of Medicine. 17 Nov. 2004 <PMID: 12019587>.

Mercier, L. R. "Epicondylitis." *Ferri's Clinical Advisor: Instant Diagnosis and Treatment.* Ed. Fred Ferri. St. Louis: Mosby-Year Book, Inc., 2000. 384. *MD Consult.*Elsevier, Inc. 5 Oct. 2004 <http://home.mdconsult.com>.

Nirschl, R. P., et al. "Iontophoretic Administration of Dexamethasone Sodium Phosphate for Acute Epicondylitis. A Randomized, Double-Blinded, Placebo-Controlled Study." *American Journal of Sports Medicine* 31 2 (2003): 189–195. *National Center for Biotechnology Information.*National Library of Medicine. 17 Nov. 2004 <PMID: 12642251>.

Smidt, N., et al. "Corticosteroid Injections, Physiotherapy, or a Wait-and-See Policy for Lateral Epicondylitis: A Randomised Controlled Trial." *Lancet* 359 9307 (2002): 657–662. *National Center for Biotechnology Information.*National Library of Medicine. 17 Nov. 2004 <PMID: 11879861>.

Smidt, N., et al. "Effectiveness of Physiotherapy for Lateral Epicondylitis: A Systematic Review." *Annals of Medicine* 35 1 (2003): 51–62. *National Center for Biotechnology Information.*National Library of Medicine. 17 Nov. 2004 <PMID: 12693613>.

Young, Craig C. "Medial Epicondylitis." *eMedicine.com.* Eds. Anthony J. Saglimbeni, et al. 26 Oct. 2004.eMedicine.com, Inc. 8 Feb. 2005 <http://www.emedicine.com/sports/topic74.htm>.

Rotator Cuff Tear

Duration | Trends | Rehabilitation | Codes | UMK | Costs | Go ... | Bookmark | Print

Related Terms: Tear of the Rotator Cuff Definition

Rotator cuff tear occurs when the tendons that form the rotator cuff weaken and tear.

The rotator cuff comprises four muscles and their tendon attachments that wrap over the upper arm (humeral head) in the shoulder. These tendons come under stress from repeated activities that require lifting and rotating the arm. Any abnormalities of the shoulder joint can aggravate the stress, especially looseness (laxity); narrowing of the impingement interval, which is the space between the shoulder blade and the collarbone (impingement syndrome); and bursitis. As the tendons become irritated, they become inflamed and eventually weaken and may tear.

Tears are described as either partial thickness tears or complete rupture, depending on the amount of tissue damage. Partial tears do not go all the way through the cuff, although there may be a fairly large surface area involved. Complete tears create a hole in the cuff with partial or total loss of tendon function. The size of tear ranges from small to massive, depending on the size of the hole created and how much of the humeral head is exposed.

Tears are classified as acute or chronic, depending on onset. Acute tears are the result of forceful injury to the shoulder and straining the tendon beyond its limits, which causes a tear. Chronic tears come from repetitive wear and tear to the cuff mechanism. Conditions that may lead to rotator cuff tear include impingement syndrome (see rotator cuff syndrome), instability of the glenohumeral joint, or inborn (congenital) abnormalities of the shoulder.

Risk: Although rotator cuff tears can affect young adults, typically as the result of a trauma, they are most often found in individuals over 40 years of age (Roy). Individuals at a higher risk of sustaining a rotator cuff tear include those who perform overhead work (e.g., warehouse workers, laborers, carpenters, construction workers) and certain athletes (e.g., swimmers, tennis players, baseball players). Men are twice as likely as women to sustain rotator cuff tears (Tuite).

Incidence and Prevalence: Rotator cuff tears may affect from 5% to 40% of the population (Malanga). In general, tears are more common in older age groups than younger ones. Cadaver studies showed that 39% of individuals over the age of 60 have full-thickness tears (Malanga), although tears may produce no symptoms, making frequency estimates difficult to verify.

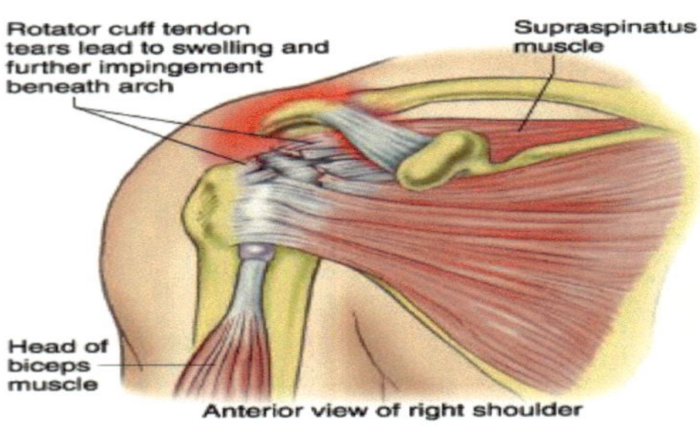

- **Diagnosis**

  History: Most individuals with acute tears will describe a fall or attempt to break a fall by grabbing a rail, or an athletic injury. Those with a chronic tear will describe increasing pain and difficulty using the shoulder. Individuals will complain of increasing shoulder pain with activity and pain at night with inability to sleep on the affected shoulder. They may complain of shoulder weakness and the inability or limited ability to raise (abduct) their arm. The individual may report that he or she has impingement syndrome.

  Physical exam: Range of shoulder motion is tested by asking individuals to raise their arm away from their side toward the ear (abduction). A tear is indicated when an individual cannot perform this maneuver or, when the arm is raised by someone else, cannot hold the position. Touching (palpation) over the top of the shoulder into the deltoid will produce pain. There may be wasting (atrophy) of the cuff muscles with fairly good range of motion (ROM) by substitution of other shoulder muscles. There are numerous other active and passive shoulder physical examination tests. Each is specific for different muscle groups and function of the shoulder. The nonaffected shoulder is examined first to establish a normal baseline.

  Tests: Plain x-rays are not diagnostic for rotator cuff tears but will show abnormalities in the bone, shoulder structure, and inflammation and calcification of the shoulder bursa (calcific tendinitis). Arthrography, MRI, or CT scan, often with contrast media (CT-arthrography), are the tests used most often to define a tear. Ultrasonography is used in many facilities, although differentiating a partial and full thickness tear may not be as accurate as with the other tests. Diagnostic arthroscopy is occasionally done to evaluate the rotator cuff and shoulder mechanics, especially on acute tears in athletes.

- **Treatment**

  The goals of treatment are pain relief and improved shoulder function. Partial tears that do not cause dramatic or progressive shoulder weakness are treated conservatively with rest, ice, NSAIDs, and, possibly local anesthetic or corticosteroid injection into the subacromial space. Physical therapy will help increase cuff strength, stabilize the shoulder blade (scapula), increase motion, and decrease pain and inflammation. Use of heat on an inflamed or torn tendon may increase pain and worsen the situation. Although nonoperative treatment will not repair the tear, it often achieves the goals of pain relief and partial restoration of function.

  Complete tears and any tears that cause marked pain or weakness and interfere with daily activities in younger adults are treated with surgical repair, either arthroscopically or with open surgery (open rotator cuff repair). Partial tears are sometimes cleaned (débrided) arthroscopically to remove the inflamed tissue and ragged edges of the tear. Rotator cuff surgery may be performed under regional or general anesthesia. Treatment in older individuals is based on overall health, weakness of the shoulder joint, pain, and the ability to function. Surgery is done to repair the tear when there are marked changes in these parameters. Otherwise, a complete tear in an elderly individual is treated conservatively, or with simpler procedures such as arthroscopic débridement and subacromial decompression. Massive tears may be inoperable and would also be treated nonoperatively.

- **Prognosis**

  Conservative treatment of small rotator cuff tears has a good outcome (a return to normal functioning) for 40% to 90% of individuals (Felsenstein) but may take 6 months or longer. Younger individuals are more likely to have a good outcome than older individuals. However, athletes have a poorer outcome in terms of returning to previous levels of competition, especially after a full-thickness rotator cuff tear. Conservative treatment of chronic, larger tears, especially in the dominant shoulder, has a poor outcome. Surgical repair of a rotator cuff tear has a good outcome in about 90% of cases (Felsenstein), provided the tear is small, there are no complications, and the individual's general health is good. Surgical repair in elderly individuals has a poor outcome, due to pre-existing rotator cuff degeneration. Massive tears have a poorer prognosis and are associated with a high degree of disability. Some individuals never regain full motion or strength in the affected shoulder.

- **Utilization Management Knowledgebase**

  SH501 Rotator Cuff Tear
  SH515 Labral Tear

- **Differential Diagnoses**

  Cervical nerve root injury
  Impingement syndrome
  Painful arc syndrome
  Rotator cuff tendinitis
  Subacromial bursitis
  Subscapular nerve entrapment

- **Specialists**

  Occupational Therapist
  Orthopedic (Orthopaedic) Surgeon
  Physiatrist
  Physical Therapist
  Rheumatologist
  Sports Medicine Internist

- **Rehabilitation**

  Note on research and authorship

  Acute Phase: The early goals of rehabilitation in the acute phase of a rotator cuff tear are to decrease pain and inflammation, to reduce the stress on the torn tendon(s), and to prevent the development of joint stiffness, which can severely complicate recovery (Kelley).

  In conjunction with pharmacological management, the individual will be instructed in the use of cold treatments to the shoulder to decrease inflammation. Reduction of stress to the healing tendon(s) is often achieved through education, ergonomic adjustments, and/or work modifications aimed at reducing painful activities (Breazeale; Mantone). Such activities often include positions in which the elbow is raised above the level of the shoulder, and should be avoided. Stiffness may be prevented by passive range of motion exercises conducted during supervised rehabilitation and a home exercise program (Mantone).

Healing Phase: As the pain and inflammation ease, treatment aims at improving strength and flexibility to the shoulder without irritating the healing tendon(s) (Breazeale). The strengthening exercises begin with scapular muscles. These are important muscles for normal shoulder function, and the exercises can usually be performed without excessively stressing the healing tendon(s). Gentle stretching exercises may be initiated, avoiding stress on the healing tendon(s). As the tendon heals, strengthening exercises are added, as indicated (Mantone).

Chronic Phase: The goal of rehabilitation in this phase is to restore pain-free function (Mantone). Strengthening exercises emphasize all muscles of the shoulder area. Flexibility exercises and manual therapy are incorporated within the available range of motion. Individuals who are not able to regain function or control pain may be evaluated for surgery.

If managed operatively, see Rotator Cuff Repair.

FREQUENCY OF REHABILITATION VISITS

Nonsurgical (Acute Phase)	
Specialist	Rotator Cuff Tear
Physical or Occupational Therapist	Up to 16 visits within 8 weeks
Surgical (Acute Phase)	
Specialist	Rotator Cuff Tear
Physical or Occupational Therapist	Up to 24 visits within 12 weeks

The table above represents a range of the usual acceptable number of visits for uncomplicated cases. It provides a framework based on the duration of tissue healing time and standard clinical practice.

- **Comorbid Conditions**

  Diabetes mellitus
  Osteoarthritis
  Osteoporosis
  Rheumatoid arthritis
  Shoulder trauma
  Tendinitis

- **Complications**

  Post-traumatic arthritis of the shoulder, impingement syndrome, osteoporosis of the humeral head, chronic inflammation of the subacromial bursa, nerve injury, frozen shoulder (adhesive capsulitis), and poor shoulder motion are possible complications.

- **Factors Influencing Duration**

  The size of the tear; the individual's age, occupation, and overall health; dominant side involvement, the need for surgery, and the effectiveness of rehabilitation may affect the length of disability. There may be permanent disability regarding certain activities. The larger the tear, the more likely that permanent weakness will result. Therefore, heavy or very heavy work may no longer be possible.

- **Length of Disability**

  Disability may be permanent for individuals who do heavy work or repetitive overhead work.

Medical treatment, rotator cuff tear

DURATION IN DAYS

Job Classification	Minimum	Optimum	Maximum
Sedentary	1	3	4
Light	1	3	7
Medium	14	21	42
Heavy	28	42	84
Very Heavy	28	42	84

Surgical treatment, arthroscopic rotator cuff repair

DURATION IN DAYS

Job Classification	Minimum	Optimum	Maximum
Sedentary	7	10	21
Light	7	14	21
Medium	28	42	56
Heavy	56	70	112
Very Heavy	56	70	112

Surgical treatment, open rotator cuff repair

DURATION IN DAYS

Job Classification	Minimum	Optimum	Maximum
Sedentary	28	42	70
Light	28	56	84
Medium	42	84	140
Heavy	70	84	140
Very Heavy	70	84	140

- **Duration Trend from Reference Data**

DURATION TRENDS

ICD-9-CM: 840.4

Cases	Mean	Min	Max	No Lost Time	Over 6 Months
3982	68	1	329	<0.1%	7.3%

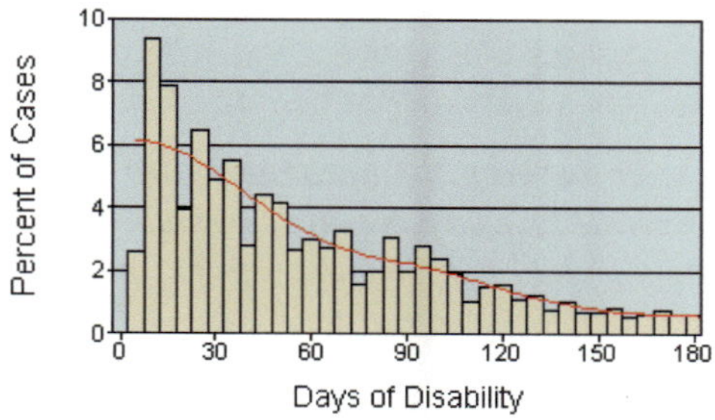

Percentile:	5th	25th	Median	75th	95th
Days:	7	21	49	96	189

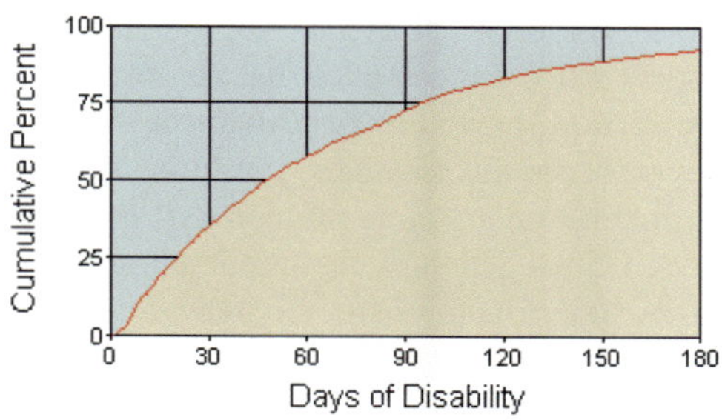

DURATION TRENDS

ICD-9-CM: 727.61

Cases	Mean	Min	Max	No Lost Time	Over 6 Months
1667	90	0	372	0.1%	10.3%

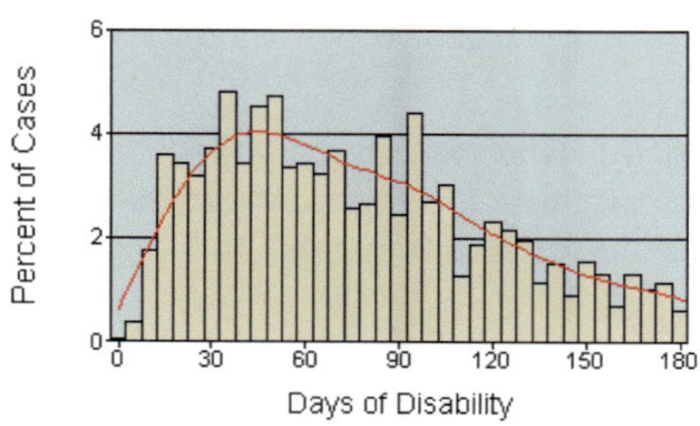

Percentile:	5th	25th	Median	75th	95th
Days:	14	42	76	123	217

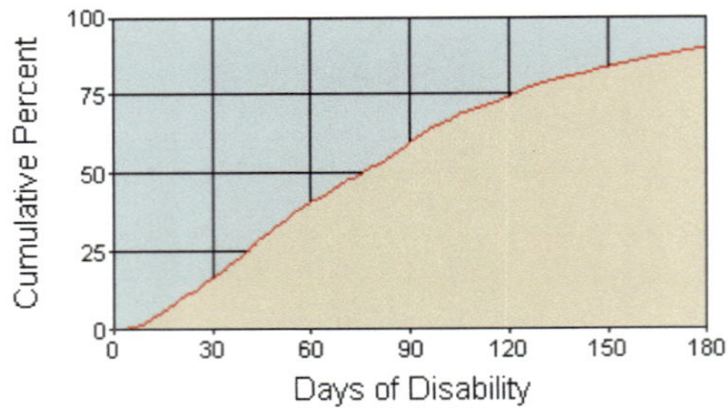

Differences may exist between the duration tables and the reference graphs. Duration tables provide expected recovery periods based on the type of work performed by the individual. The reference graphs reflect the actual experience of many individuals across the spectrum of physical conditions, in a variety of industries, and with varying levels of case management. Selected graphs combine multiple codes based on similar means and medians.

- **Return to Work (Restrictions / Accommodations)**

Limiting use of the affected shoulder or avoiding any use at all may be necessary. Arm use above shoulder level should be avoided. The arm and hand can be used at the individual's side for activities that do not require lifting, pushing, or carrying. These restrictions may become permanent. An ergonomic evaluation of the workplace may be necessary. Changing job duties, sharing or alternating tasks, working at a reduced rate, taking more frequent rest breaks, and limiting the time and frequency of repetitive activities are important accommodations. Work site modifications can include forearm rests for individuals who use computer keyboards frequently, headsets for those who answer telephones, and alterations such that repetitive activities are performed with the arms in a lower level of elevation.

Recovery from surgical repair is the most restrictive, with no use of the arm and shoulder for 2 months and only a gradual increase in allowed activities. The use of a sling will affect manual dexterity. Some individuals will never regain full range of motion or strength in the affected arm. Depending on job duties, individuals may require permanent reassignment, which may necessitate retraining. Use of analgesics and other medications can affect dexterity and alertness. Use of these medications may require review of drug policies.

- **Failure to Recover**

If an individual fails to recover within the maximum duration expectancy period, the reader may wish to reference the following questions to assist in better understanding the specifics of an individual's medical case.

Regarding diagnosis:

Does individual have any risk factors for a rotator cuff tear (those who perform overhead work, certain athletes, those who have impingement syndrome, instability of the glenohumeral joint, or congenital abnormalities of the shoulder)?

Did individual fall?

Did individual experience associated shoulder weakness or inability to raise his or her arm?

Did individual have any positive findings on exam, such as pain in the deltoid, muscle atrophy, or impairment of range of motion?

Has individual received adequate testing to establish the diagnosis (i.e., MRI, CT scan, arthroscopy)?

If diagnosis was uncertain, were other conditions with similar symptoms been ruled out (i.e., painful arc syndrome, impingement syndrome, rotator cuff tendinitis, biceps tendinitis, and subacromial bursitis)?

Regarding treatment:

Has individual responded favorably to conservative treatment of rest, ice, NSAIDs, and physical therapy? If not, have steroid injections been tried?

Did it become necessary to repair the tear surgically?

Regarding prognosis:

Is individual active in physical therapy? Does the individual have a home exercise program?

Is individual's employer able to accommodate necessary restrictions?

Is affected shoulder on the dominant or nondominant side?

Does individual have any other conditions, such as shoulder dislocation or other shoulder injuries, osteoarthritis, rheumatoid arthritis, diabetes, gout, or osteoporosis, that could affect recovery?

Has individual experienced any complications that could affect recovery and prognosis?

- **Medical Codes**

ICD-9-CM: 718.01, 727.61, 840.4
ICD-10: S43.4, S43.7

- **Cited References**

Breazeale, N. M., and E. V. Craig. "Partial-Thickness Rotator Cuff Tears. Pathogenesis and Treatment." *Orthopedic Clinics of North America* 28 2 (1997): 145–155. *National Center for Biotechnology Information*.National Library of Medicine. 14 Dec. 2004 <PMID: 9113711>.

Felsenstein, Chad H., and Robert M. McNamara. "Rotator Cuff Injury." *eMedicine Consumer Health*. Eds. Scott H. Plantz, et al. 7 Sep. 2004.eMedicine.com, Inc. 29 Oct. 2004 <http://www.emedicinehealth.com/articles/5582-1.asp>.

Kelley, M. J., and William A. Clark, eds. *Orthopedic Therapy of the Shoulder*. Philadelphia : J.B. Lippincott Company, 1995.

Malanga, Gerard A. "Rotator Cuff Injury." *eMedicine.com*. Eds. Andrew L. Sherman, et al. 17 Dec. 2004.eMedicine.com, Inc. 29 Oct. 2004 <http://www.emedicine.com/sports/topic115.htm>.

Mantone, J. K., W. Z. Burkhead, and J. Noonan. “Nonoperative Treatment of Rotator Cuff Tears.” *Orthopedic Clinics of North America* 31 2 (2000): 295–311. *National Center for Biotechnology Information*.National Library of Medicine. 14 Dec. 2004 <PMID: 10736398>.

Roy, Andre. “Rotator Cuff Disease.” *eMedicine.com*. Eds. Robert E. Windsor, et al. 12 Jan. 2005.eMedicine.com, Inc. 29 Oct. 2004 <http://www.emedicine.com/pmr/topic125.htm>.

Tuite, Michael. “Shoulder, Rotator Cuff Injury (MRI).” *eMedicine.com*. Eds. David S. Levey, et al. 7 Jul. 2004.eMedicine.com, Inc. 29 Oct. 2004 <http://www.emedicine.com/radio/topic894.htm>.

Tendinitis

Duration | Trends | Rehabilitation | Codes | UMK | Costs   Go ... | Bookmark | Print

Related Terms: Tendonitis

- **Definition**

Tendinitis is inflammation of a tendon, the fibrous tissue that connects a muscle to bone. Some tendons are rope-like and others are similar to thick sheets. The inflammation is often accompanied by degeneration of the collagen fibers comprising the tendon.

Tendinitis occurs only when there is direct injury to the tendon itself along with partial tearing of the fibers. Tendinitis is a very common condition, prevalent in individuals engaged in sporting events and/or heavy labor. Tendinitis can be caused from an infection, acute trauma, poor technique with activity, lack of strength and flexibility, age-related deterioration, or overload or overuse of the affected tendon. The condition can also be caused by inflammatory diseases such as rheumatoid arthritis, systemic sclerosis, gout, Reiter’s syndrome, and diabetes mellitus.

Inflamed tendons are frequently found in the hand. Other common sites for tendinitis are in the shoulder and knee (rotator cuff tendinitis, patellar tendinitis, and iliotibial band tendinitis). Tendinitis that affects the site of tendon insertion into the bone (insertional tendinopathy) is the most common. Since tendons fail to regenerate quickly because of lack of a rich blood supply, aging may also cause gradual deterioration (tendinosis). The term “tendinosis” is used to describe the chronically painful degenerative tendon. In this condition there are no inflammatory cells present, unlike acute tendinitis.

Calcific tendinitis occurs when calcium deposits form in the tendons, usually at the rotator cuff. This type of tendinitis will frequently resolve spontaneously in 1 to 4 weeks (Cluett).

Ongoing (chronic) conditions result from microtrauma or “overuse” of the tendon, with symptoms developing over time. The overuse can be caused from excessive pressure or workload. Tendon failure occurs from stretching of collagen fibers within the tendon. Up to 4% of tendon elongation is tolerated well; however, from 4% to 8% of tendon elongation causes microtrauma, and greater than 8% of tendon elongation causes macrotrauma with rupture of the tendon fibers (Rettig). Repetitive tasks and excessive exercise also may cause tendinitis. Shearing stress on the tendon may occur where tendons pass in close proximity to the bone. Sudden onset (acute) or traumatic tendinitis may be caused by a bruise with bleeding into the tissue (contusion) or muscle-tendon strain.

Risk: Tendinitis is generally most common in males, and Achilles tendon tears occur 4 to 7 times more frequently in males than females (Maffulli). Individuals who are middle-aged are more likely to develop tendinitis (Steele). Calcific tendinitis usually occurs in individuals between the ages of 30 to 40, and is more frequent in those who are diabetic (Cluett).

Incidence and Prevalence: Incidence of tendinitis as an occupational injury is 11 per 100,000 individuals who work full-time ("Incidence Rates").

Overuse tendinitis is most common in the wrist and hand, and comprises between 25% to 50% of all sports injuries (Rettig).

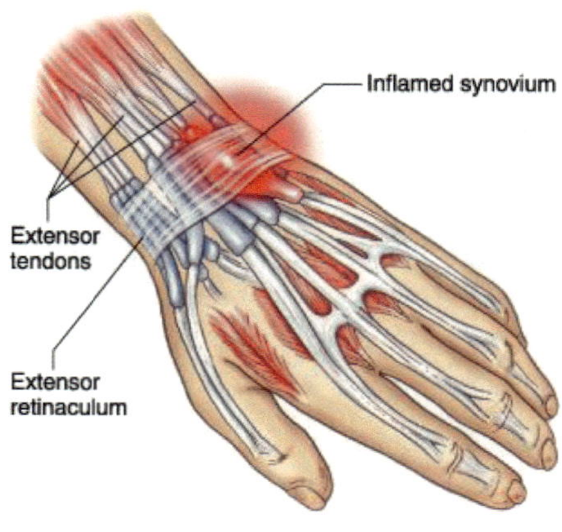

- **Diagnosis**

History: Individuals with tendinitis caused by trauma may have heard or felt a "pop" as the tendon fibers tore. There may be increasing pain. Most individuals, however, report symptoms that begin gradually. Ongoing (chronic) tendinitis creates symptoms including pain during or after activity. Other symptoms may include swelling, stiffness and a sensation of creaking or squeaking with motion.

Individuals with tendinitis of the hand caused by infection may report pain and swelling over the top (dorsum) of the hand. There may be history of a recent bacterial infection, an open wound, or tuberculosis. Individuals may also report previous injuries that may not have been successfully diagnosed and rehabilitated.

Physical exam: Swelling, warmth and tenderness may be evident. A stethoscopic exam may reveal creaking or popping (crepitus) noises along the course of the tendon. Pain accompanying movement may be detected. There may be a visible deformity, such as a torn biceps tendon curling and making a ball under the skin. A neurovascular exam may be necessary to rule out compartment syndrome and nerve injury.

Tests: An x-ray may reveal calcium deposits along the tendon and sheath. MRI may be needed to identify tendon tears. Laboratory studies, x-ray, bone scans, and compartment pressure measurements may be used to rule out complications or underlying conditions.

- **Treatment**

  Tendinitis caused by trauma, especially if it occurs suddenly (acute), is generally treated with rest, ice (cold therapy), compressive dressing and elevation to control swelling (RICE). Heat rather than cold therapy might be used for acute forms of the condition, depending on patient response. Nonsteroidal anti-inflammatory drugs (NSAIDs) are prescribed for pain and swelling. Muscle-tendon length should be maintained with gentle stretching. When the onset (acute) episode has passed, rehabilitation for strengthening may be needed to prevent re-injury.

  Ongoing (chronic) tendinitis is treated by stopping the aggravating activity, RICE, NSAIDs and physical therapy to control pain and swelling. With the chronic form, heat may be more effective than cold in therapy. Muscle strengthening may be recommended to restore normal function.

  Corticosteroids and/or anesthetics may be injected into the tendon sheath to relieve pain and swelling. In extreme cases, surgery (excision, tenosynovectomy) may be needed to remove inflamed tissue or calcium deposits. Ruptured tendons may require repair through suturing (ruptured tendon repair).

- **Prognosis**

  Full recovery is likely to occur in ongoing (chronic) cases. In severe cases, traumatic tendinitis with rupture may require surgery (ruptured tendon repair) and take longer to heal. Tendinitis in the hand caused by infection (infective tendinitis) can lead to loss of tendon structure. Repair of the tendon, excision, or tenosynovectomy will likely have a good outcome if damage to the tendon is not extensive. Cases requiring surgery are rare, but individuals with significant tendon damage may experience at least partial loss of function. The recovery period also is likely to be painful.

- **Utilization Management Knowledgebase**

  ANF501 Ankle or Foot Tendinitis
  ELB509 Tendonitis
  KN512 Patellar Tendinitis

- **Differential Diagnoses**

  Bursitis
  Carpal tunnel syndrome

Chronic compartment syndrome
Distal nerve compression injury
Myositis ossificans
Radiculitis
Rheumatoid arthritis
Stress fracture
Vascular disorders

- **Specialists**

Internal Medicine Physician
Orthopedic (Orthopaedic) Surgeon
Physiatrist
Rheumatologist
Sports Medicine Internist

- **Rehabilitation**

Note on research and authorship

The initial goals of rehabilitation for tendinitis are controlling pain and swelling, followed by regaining motion, flexibility, strength, and endurance of the tendon, muscle, and involved joint structures. An effort should be made to identify the underlying cause of the current symptoms, after which, when possible, modifications should be made to reduce the risk factors associated with the condition.

Modalities such as heat and cold may be used throughout rehabilitation to control pain and swelling (Braddom). If pain significantly limits motion, then splinting the involved part may be necessary. When indicated, therapy should begin with range of motion exercises, progress to strengthening exercises as indicated, and continue by instructing individuals in a home exercise program to complement supervised rehabilitation (Biundo; Mafi).

The final goal is returning the individual to full function for work and recreational activities with minimal risk of re-injury. If work tasks expose the individual to risk factors for tendinitis, an ergonomic assessment may be indicated. If leisure activities are suspect, the individual should be educated in ways to modify the activity and decrease the likelihood of developing symptoms.

Additional information may provide insight into the rehabilitation needs of these individuals (Huang).

FREQUENCY OF REHABILITATION VISITS

Nonsurgical	
Specialist	Tendinitis
Physical, Occupational or Hand Therapist	Up to 16 visits within 8 weeks

The table above represents a range of the usual acceptable number of visits for uncomplicated cases. It provides a framework based on the duration of tissue healing time and standard clinical practice.

- **Comorbid Conditions**

Diabetes mellitus
Rheumatoid arthritis

- **Complications**

  Compartment syndrome and nerve injury may be caused by tissue swelling associated with tendinitis. Inflammation of the lining of the tendon sheath (tenosynovitis) often accompanies tendinitis, and may occur with infection by gonococcal bacteria that is transmitted sexually (gonorrhea). When tendinitis is treated with corticosteroid injections, cell death and tendon atrophy may result. Tendon rupture may occur. When tendon fibers are torn away from the bone, usually from excessive pulling forces, the result is a condition called enthesopathy. Inflammation in tendons of the hand may cause the thumb to extend (de Quervain's disease). Fingers and/or the thumb may be hampered in movement by swelling of the tendons, which creates a sensation of popping or catching (trigger finger).

- **Factors Influencing Duration**

  Location of the tendinitis, severity, ability to control aggravating activities, treatment required, and complications might affect the disability period.

- **Length of Disability**

Medical and/or supportive treatment, tendinitis.

DURATION IN DAYS

Job Classification	Minimum	Optimum	Maximum
Sedentary	1	3	7
Light	1	7	14
Medium	3	14	56
Heavy	3	21	56
Very Heavy	3	28	56

- **Duration Trend from Reference Data**

DURATION TRENDS

ICD-9-CM: 726.9, 726.90					
Cases	Mean	Min	Max	No Lost Time	Over 6 Months
1256	41	0	204	0.4%	2.6%

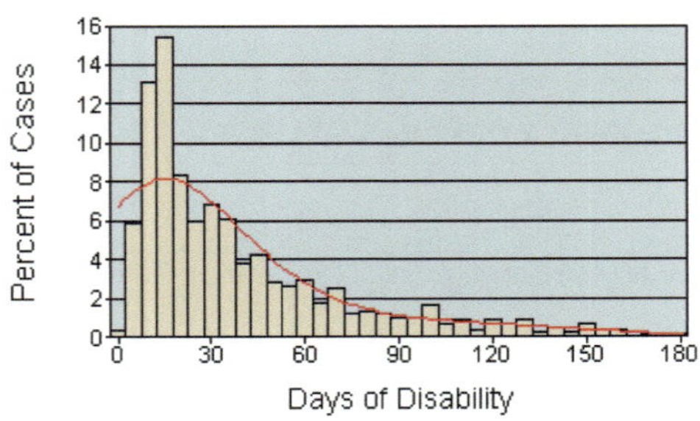

Percentile:	5th	25th	Median	75th	95th
Days:	4	12	26	54	134

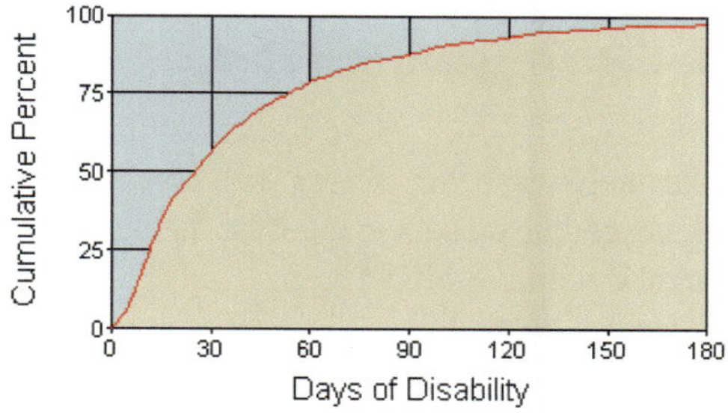

Differences may exist between the duration tables and the reference graphs. Duration tables provide expected recovery periods based on the type of work performed by the individual. The reference graphs reflect the actual experience of many individuals across the spectrum of physical conditions, in a variety of industries, and with varying levels of case management. Selected graphs combine multiple codes based on similar means and medians.

- **Return to Work (Restrictions / Accommodations)**

Restrictions include removing aggravating activities, depending on the tendon involved. This may include avoidance of lifting, carrying, twisting movements of the wrist or forearm, repetitive and overhead work. Use of protective or assistive devices such as splints, crutches, or slings may affect dexterity. Safety issues may need to be evaluated. Prescribed medication for control of symptoms may require review of drug policies.

Return to work requiring physical activity may need monitoring, as many individuals attempt to resume "normal" activity too soon. This often leads to a cycle of re-injuries.

Failure to Recover

If an individual fails to recover within the maximum duration expectancy period, the reader may wish to reference the following questions to assist in better understanding the specifics of an individual's medical case.

Regarding diagnosis:

Does individual have a history of injury, overload, or overuse of the tendon?

Does individual have a history of rheumatoid arthritis, systemic sclerosis, gout, Reiter's syndrome, or diabetes mellitus?

Does individual's work or play involve repetitive tasks or excessive exercise?

Which tendon is involved?

Does individual report hearing a pop with injury?

Does individual report a gradual onset of pain during or after activity, swelling, stiffness and a sensation of creaking or squeaking with motion?

On exam, was swelling, warmth, tenderness, or crepitus evident?

Is pain with movement detected? Is there visible deformity?

Has individual had an x-ray, MRI, bone scan or compartment pressure measurements?

Was neurovascular exam necessary?

Have conditions with similar symptoms been ruled out?

Regarding treatment:

Is individual with an acute injury being treated with rest, ice, compression and elevation (RICE)? Is heat, depending on patient response, being used rather than ice?

Is individual being treated with NSAIDs?

Has physical therapy been prescribed?

Has individual stopped aggravating activity?

Has individual received an injection of corticosteroids and/or anesthetics?

Did tenosynovectomy become necessary?

Was ruptured tendon repaired surgically?

Regarding prognosis:

Is individual active in physical therapy?

Does individual have a home exercise program?

Does individual have any conditions that may affect ability to recover?

Does individual have any complications such as compartment syndrome, nerve injury tenosynovitis, tendon rupture, enthesopathy, de Quervain's disease or a trigger finger?

- **Medical Codes**

ICD-9-CM:	726.10, 726.11, 726.61, 726.64, 726.71, 726.72, 726.79, 726.9, 726.90
ICD-10:	M25.7, M65.8, M71.5, M77.9, M89.9

- **Cited References**

Biundo, J. J., R. W. Irwin, and E. Umpierre. "Sports and Other Soft Tissue Injuries Tendinitis, Bursitis, and Occupation-related Syndromes." *Current Opinion in Rheumatology* 13 2 (2001): 146–149. *National Center for Biotechnology Information*.National Library of Medicine. 1 Dec. 2004 <PMID: 11224739>.

Braddom, Randolph L. *Physical Medicine and Rehabilitation.* 2nd ed. Philadelphia: W.B. Saunders, 2000.

Cluett, Jonathan. "Calcific Tendonitis." *About.com.* 21 Jan. 2004 <http://www.about.com>.

Huang, H. H., A. A. Qureshi, and J. J. Biundo. "Sports and Other Soft Tissue Injuries, Tendinitis, Bursitis, and Occupation-Related Syndromes." *Current Opinion in Rheumatology* 12 2 (2000): 150–154. *National Center for Biotechnology Information*.National Library of Medicine. 1 Dec. 2004 <PMID: 10751018>.

"Incidence Rates for Nonfatal Occupational Injuries and Illnesses Involving Days Away from Work per 10,000 Full-time Workers for Selected Characteristics and Industry Division, United States, 2002." *U.S. Department of Labor*.U.S. Department of Labor. 27 Oct. 2004 <http://www.bls.gov/opub/cwc/sh20040414tb06.htm>.

Maffulli, N., J. Wong, and L. C. Almekinders. "Types and Epidemiology of Tendinopathy." *Clinics in Sports Medicine* 22 4 (2003): 675–692. *MD Consult.* Elsevier, Inc. 27 Oct. 2004 <http://home.mdconsult.com>.

Mafi, N., R. Lorentzon, and H. Alfredson. "Superior Short-term Results with Eccentric Calf Muscle Training Compared to Concentric Training in a

Randomized Prospective Multicenter Study on Patients with Chronic Achilles Tendinosis." *Knee Surgery, Sports Traumatology, Arthroscopy* 9 1 (2001): 42–47. *National Center for Biotechnology Information*.National Library of Medicine. 1 Dec. 2004 <PMID: 11269583>.

Rettig, A. C. "Wrist and Hand Overuse Syndromes." *Clinics in Sports Medicine* 20 3 (2001): 591–611. *MD Consult*.Elsevier, Inc. 27 Oct. 2004 <http://home.mdconsult.com>.

Steele, Mark. "Tendonitis." *eMedicine.com*. Eds. Richard S. Krause, et al. 11 Nov. 2004.eMedicine.com, Inc. 27 Oct. 2004 <http://www.emedicine.com/emerg/topic570.htm>.

Depression, Major

Duration | Trends | Codes | Costs   Go ... | Bookmark | Print

Related Terms: Depressive Psychosis, Major Depressive Disorder, Psychotic Depression, Unipolar Depression

- **Definition**

Major depression is a serious psychiatric illness that negatively affects how an individual feels, thinks, and acts. Everyone experiences depressed moods as a result of a change, either in the form of a setback or a loss, or as Freud said, "everyday misery." The sadness and depressed feelings that accompany the changes and losses of life are usually appropriate, necessary, transitory, and can present an opportunity for personal growth. However, depression that persists and results in serious dysfunction in daily life could be an indication of a depressive disorder that may need to be treated as a medical problem. Severity, duration, and presence of other symptoms are factors that distinguish normal sadness from a depressive disorder.

Major depression, called major depressive disorder in the DSM-IV-TR (Diagnostic and Statistical Manual of Mental Disorders, 4th Edition, Text Revision), is a mood disorder distinguished by the occurrence of one or more major depressive episodes. A major depressive episode is diagnosed when an individual experiences persistent feelings of sadness or anxiety, with loss of interest or pleasure in usual activities (anhedonia). In addition, five or more of the following symptoms must be present for at least two consecutive weeks: changes in appetite that result in weight losses or gains not related to dieting; insomnia or oversleeping; loss of energy or increased fatigue; restlessness or irritability; feelings of worthlessness or inappropriate guilt; difficulty thinking, concentrating, or making decisions; and thoughts of death or suicide, or attempts at suicide.

A depressive episode is diagnosed only if the above symptoms are not due to any other psychiatric conditions (such as bipolar disorder) or medical conditions (such as neurological or hormonal problems, cancer, or heart attack). Symptoms must not be due to unexpected side effects of medications or substance abuse.

The DSM-IV-TR divides major depressive disorder into two subtypes based on whether or not the individual has experienced a single depressive episode or recurrent depressive episodes. The DSM-IV-TR also adds specifiers to a diagnosis, rating severity along a continuum of mild, moderate, severe, and severe with psychotic features. The latter is sometimes known as depressive psychosis. Partial and full remissions are additional specifiers.

Major depression can afflict anyone, regardless of age, race, class, or sex. Only a third of depressed individuals receive proper treatment. Recently, a study showed that of bereaved spouses who meet major depression criteria, 83% received no antidepressant medication. One explanation for the low percentage of treatment of depressed individuals is that society has stigmatized mental illness for so long that people with depression, and sometimes their families, feel too ashamed to acknowledge the disease and to seek treatment.

It is estimated that up to 25% of individuals experiencing severe medical conditions will experience a concurrent major depressive disorder (DSM-IV-TR 372-73).

Risk: Major risk factors are female sex, age, family history, bereavement, and brain injury. Women suffer from the disorder at least twice as often as men in societies around the world. The peak age at onset is between 20 and 25 years, and 40 and 45 years. Although older individuals frequently seek treatment, there is no evidence that major depression is more common in older than in younger adults. Individuals who have parents or siblings with major depression have a 1.5 to 3 times greater risk of developing this disorder. Grief is a risk factor because it may turn into major depression, especially in bereaved spouses, who often meet the criteria for major depression.

Incidence and Prevalence: In the US, lifetime risk is 10% to 25% for women, and 5% to 12% for men. An international study (17 researchers, 38,000 individuals from 10 countries) reported that the lifetime risk of depression ranged from 1.5% in Taiwan to 19% in Lebanon. Risks in other countries, in ascending order, were 2.9% in Korea, 4.3% in Puerto Rico, 5.2% in the US, 9.2% in Germany, 9.6% in Canada, 11.6% in New Zealand, and 16.4% in France.

- **Diagnosis**

History: A thorough history includes taking an account of current and previous symptoms, questions about mood, memory, and changes in relationships, and corroborative history from friends, family members, or employers. It is important to determine whether there is a family history of depression or of suicides. A careful, non-judgmental inventory of substance abuse should be made in every case, as this requires specific treatment measures of its own. A general history of psychological problems could predispose an individual to depression. Because physical conditions have been associated with depression, a thorough history should include an account of diseases such as neurologic disorders (stroke, Parkinson's, and Alzheimer's disease, multiple sclerosis, epilepsy, encephalitis, brain tumors); endocrine disorders (diabetes mellitus, hypothyroidism, and hyperparathyroidism); and other disorders (coronary artery disease, cancer, and chronic fatigue syndrome). Conversely, individuals with major depression may see a medical doctor for physical complaints of headache, abdominal pain, body aches, low energy, feeling poorly, or problems with sexual function.

It is also important to obtain a complete drug history because major depression has been shown to be a side effect of some medications, especially antihypertensive agents (such as calcium channel and beta blockers), analgesics, and certain migraine medicines.

Physical exam: Complete physical examination and medical workup are indicated to rule out medical causes. Illnesses that frequently cause depression include hyperthyroidism and other glandular disturbances, cancer, stroke, and heart attack. As these illnesses are usually associated with dramatic symptoms, individuals are likely to have already sought medical attention. When the disease process is less acute and without many outward signs, however, depression may be the only complaint.

Tests: Besides routine laboratory tests, more specialized endocrine tests may be helpful in establishing the diagnosis. A CT may also be requested to test for relatively rare causes such as brain tumor or a clinically silent stroke. Psychological tests such as the Minnesota Multiphasic Personality Inventory - 2 (MMPI-2) and the Beck Depression Inventory (BDI) may be useful in establishing a baseline of reported symptoms and monitoring response to treatment.

- **Treatment**

Treatment choice depends on the outcome of the evaluation (history, physical exam, and tests). Treatment usually consists of psychotherapy, medications, or both. Today, there are a number of effective antidepressant medications that work by correcting imbalances in the levels of brain chemicals (neurotransmitters). About two-thirds of individuals treated will respond to one or more medications. Generally, these medications take full effect 3 to 6 weeks after treatment has begun. Psychiatrists usually recommend that individuals continue to take the medication for five or more months after symptoms have improved.

Treatment of depression consists of three phases. Acute treatment, lasting 6 to 12 weeks, is aimed at remission of symptoms. Continuation treatment, lasting 4 to 9 months, is aimed at preventing relapse. During this phase, medication should be continued at full dosage. Psychotherapy may also be helpful. Maintenance treatment is aimed at preventing new episodes (recurrence) in individuals with prior episodes. Both maintenance medication and maintenance psychotherapy can prevent relapse or delay the next episode. Individuals and their families should be educated before treatment about the diagnosis, likely outcome, treatment options, costs, and side effects.

Psychotherapy or talk therapy may be used alone for treatment of mild depression. Antidepressant medications in combination with psychotherapy are used for moderate to major depression. Different types of psychotherapy include cognitive-behavioral therapy, psychodynamic psychotherapy, interpersonal therapy, and supportive psychotherapy. In a major analysis of four randomized comparative studies, cognitive-behavioral therapy was shown to be as effective as antidepressants in treating severe or major depression, but not dysthymia.

Much of the success of psychologic therapy, in any case, depends on the skill of the therapist.

Research indicates that using a combination of antidepressants and therapy is more effective than either treatment alone for most individuals, possibly because most individuals are more likely to take their medication regularly when they are also undergoing therapy.

For those for whom neither medications nor psychotherapy are effective, other techniques, such as electroconvulsive therapy (ECT), are safe and effective. Although ECT has received bad press since it was introduced in the 1930s, it has been refined over the years, and is now successful in treating more than 90% of individuals suffering from mood disorders.

Psychiatric hospitalization is warranted in instances when there is indication of personal neglect or high-risk of self-harm.

- **Prognosis**

Most individuals with a major depressive episode will get better. As the number of available antidepressant medications continues to grow, most individuals will respond to at least one of these. Individual may also benefit from psychotherapy. With time, recovery is usually complete, though risk of relapse increases with each episode. More than half of all individuals with one episode of major depression will have another, while those individuals with a history of three previous episodes have a 90% likelihood of having a fourth. Because of this high relapse rate, it is now recommended that individuals with a history of multiple depressive episodes receive medication for the rest of their lives.

Spontaneous recovery may take months. During that time the individual is at such a great risk of complications that it would be unthinkable not to intervene. Risk of recurrence is about 70% at 5 years, and at least 80% at 8 years. For individuals with severe major depression, 76% on antidepressants recover, whereas only 18% on sugar pills (placebo) or on psychotherapy without medication recover.

Poor outcome is associated with inadequate treatment, severe initial symptoms (including psychosis), early age of onset, greater number of previous episodes, only partial recovery after 1 year, having another severe mental or medical disorder, and family dysfunction.

Major depression causes more physical and social dysfunction than many chronic medical conditions.

- **Differential Diagnoses**

Adjustment disorder with depressed mood
Bipolar disorder
Dementia
Dysthymic disorder
Mood disorder due to general condition

Schizoaffective disorder
Substance-induced mood disorder

- **Specialists**

  Clinical Psychologist | Psychiatrist

- **Comorbid Conditions**

  Alcohol/substance abuse
  Anxiety disorders
  Cardiac conditions
  Other general medical conditions
  Personality disorders

- **Complications**

  Substance abuse, especially alcohol, frequently complicates a diagnosis for depression, although in some cases it may be difficult to determine which problem is primary. About 80% to 90% of individuals with major depression also have anxiety symptoms, such as anxiety, obsessive preoccupation, panic attacks, phobias, and excessive health concerns, and about one-third also have a full-blown anxiety disorder—usually panic disorder, obsessive-compulsive disorder, or social phobia. Anxiety symptoms may require special treatment, but frequently respond to antidepressant medications, reinforcing the view that the two disorders share common brain chemistry imbalances. Approximately 1 in 10 individuals who has experienced a major depressive episode will subsequently be diagnosed as having bipolar mood disorder, a chronic condition with episodes of both depression and mania, that may only partly respond to treatment. In some cases, an episode of bipolar mood disorder may emerge as the result of antidepressant medication use.

  In extremely severe cases of major depression, psychotic symptoms may be present, such as hearing voices (auditory hallucinations) or having false beliefs (delusions).

  Up to 15% of individuals with severe major depression die by suicide. Death rate is 4 times higher over age 55. Suicide attempt may paradoxically occur as the individual begins to respond to therapy because the extreme apathy sometimes seen in major depression before treatment may actually prevent them from committing suicide due to lack of motivation or energy.

- **Factors Influencing Duration**

  Length of disability might be influenced by the severity of the illness, the presence of complicating factors such as substance abuse or suicide attempts, response to therapy, and the occupation requirements. Only in the most severe and unusual cases should this result in permanent disability.

  Substance abuse will complicate treatment and may significantly delay returning to work. Suicide attempts that lead to hospitalization will also be associated with longer periods of disability.

- **Length of Disability**

Psychotherapy and/or pharmacotherapy, major depressive disorder (single episode).

DURATION IN DAYS

Job Classification	Minimum	Optimum	Maximum
Any Work	14	28	56

Psychotherapy and/or pharmacotherapy, major depressive disorder (recurrent episode).

DURATION IN DAYS

Job Classification	Minimum	Optimum	Maximum
Any Work	14	28	70

- **Duration Trend from Reference Data**

DURATION TRENDS

ICD-9-CM: 296.2

Cases	Mean	Min	Max	No Lost Time	Over 6 Months
6347	52	0	266	2.5%	4.1%

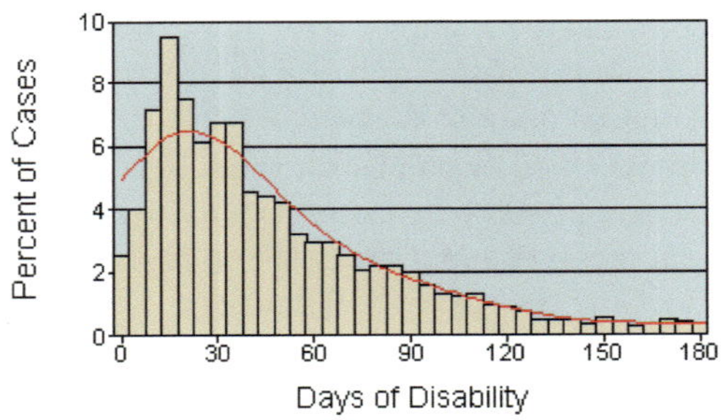

Percentile:	5th	25th	Median	75th	95th
Days:	4	17	35	71	167

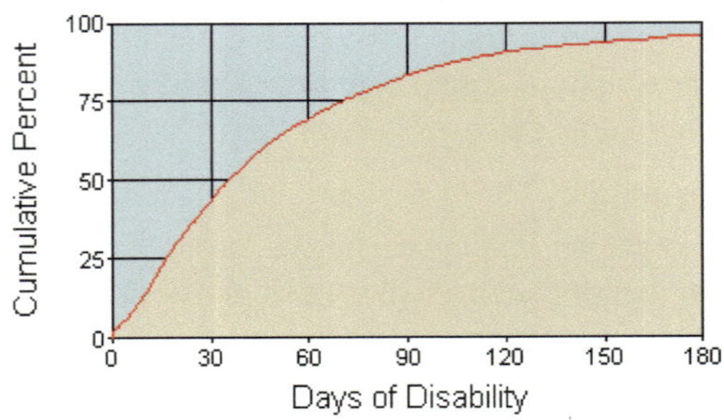

DURATION TRENDS

ICD-9-CM: 296.3, 296.32, 296.33

Cases	Mean	Min	Max	No Lost Time	Over 6 Months
3693	74	0	360	0.1%	9.2%

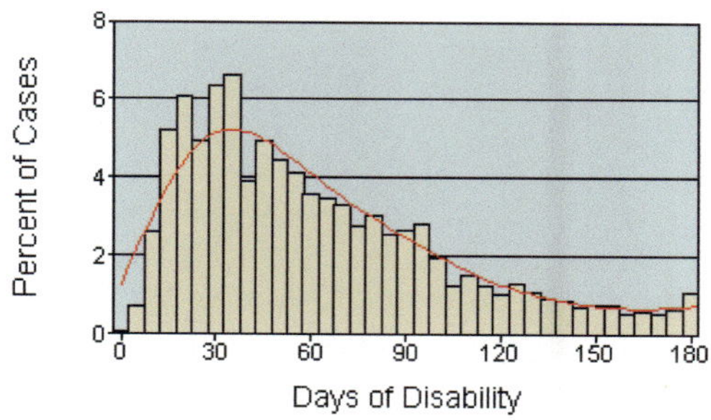

Percentile:	5th	25th	Median	75th	95th
Days:	12	30	55	97	189

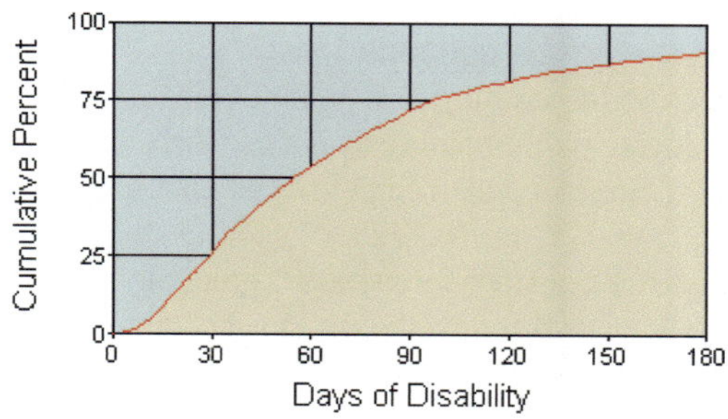

DURATION TRENDS

ICD-9-CM: 311

Cases	Mean	Min	Max	No Lost Time	Over 6 Months
9185	68	0	315	< 0.1%	8.6%

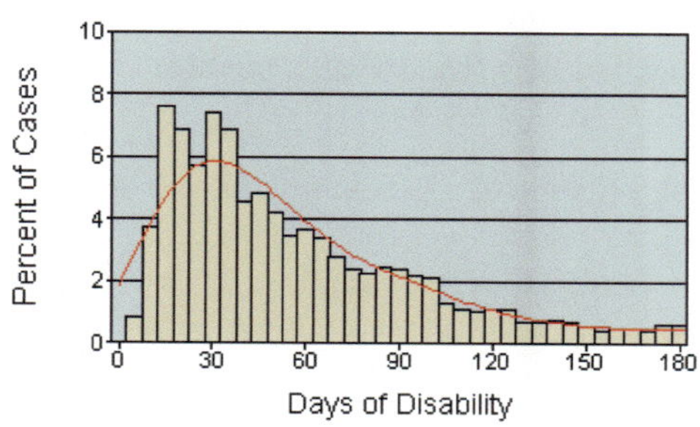

Percentile:	5th	25th	Median	75th	95th
Days:	11	26	47	90	196

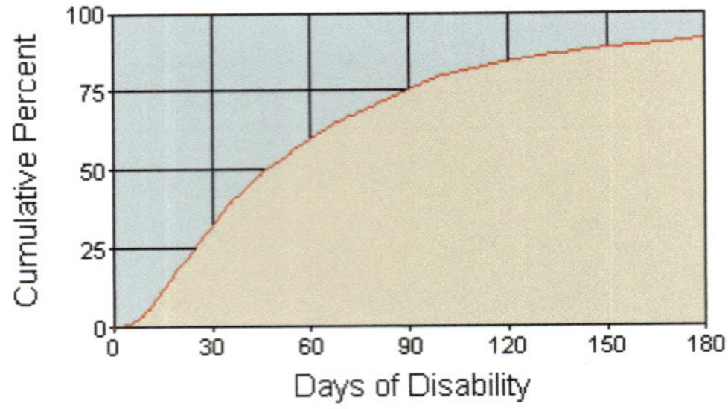

Differences may exist between the duration tables and the reference graphs. Duration tables provide expected recovery periods based on the type of work performed by the individual. The reference graphs reflect the actual experience of many individuals across the spectrum of physical conditions, in a variety of industries, and with varying levels of case management. Selected graphs combine multiple codes based on similar means and medians.

- **Return to Work (Restrictions / Accommodations)**

  Temporary work accommodations may include the avoidance of stressful situations and may include reducing or eliminating activities where the safety of self or others is contingent upon a constant and/or high level of alertness, such as driving motor vehicles, operating complex machinery, or handling dangerous chemicals; introducing the individual to new or stressful situations gradually under individually appropriate supervision; allowing some flexibility in scheduling to attend therapy appointments (which normally should occur during employee's personal time); promoting planned, proactive management of identified problem areas; and offering timely feedback on job performance issues. It will be helpful if accommodations are documented in a written plan designed to promote timely and safe transition back to full work productivity. Daytime work hours may be necessary for a period of time.

- **Failure to Recover**

  If an individual fails to recover within the maximum duration expectancy period, the reader may wish to reference the following questions to assist in better understanding the specifics of an individual's medical case.

  Regarding diagnosis:

  Was a thorough history obtained? Does family have history of depression or of suicides?

  Was substance abuse identified or ruled out?

  Does individual have history of psychological problems? Does individual have any physical conditions such as neurologic disorders (stroke, Parkinson's, epilepsy), endocrine disorders (diabetes mellitus, hypothyroidism, or hyperparathyroidism), or other disorders (cancer, coronary artery disease)?

  Were endocrine tests done?

  Is the physician an expert in diagnosis and psychopharmacology?

Was diagnosis confirmed?
Is it possible that individual was misdiagnosed?
Would individual benefit from a second opinion?

Regarding treatment:

Since major depression is the result of biochemical imbalances in the brain, is the physician adequately trained in psychopharmacology?

Even though the right medication is prescribed, does the dosage need to be increased in order to achieve an adequate level of therapeutic benefit?

Is individual beginning to feel any positive response from current medication(s)? Because responses differ and several trials of medicine may be needed before an effective treatment is found, is change of medication warranted at this time?

If individual is experiencing side effects from current medication, is individual comfortable with and diligent in reporting side effects to doctor? If not, does individual trust family member or caregiver to share this information with physician?

Is psychotherapy being used as part of individual's treatment regimen?

Is individual learning to recognize and change behaviors, thoughts, or relationships that cause or maintain depression? Is therapy helping individual to develop more healthful and rewarding habits?

Are underlying medical conditions that may complicate treatment or impact recovery being effectively addressed?

If individual's depression is incapacitating, severe and life-threatening, or if he or she cannot take or does not respond to antidepressant medications, is electroconvulsive therapy (ECT) being considered at this time?

Is individual seriously contemplating suicide or previously attempted it? Does the threat of self-harm or personal neglect put individual at risk?

Is individual frail because of weight loss or at risk for heart problems because of severe agitation?

Would individual benefit from hospitalization until self-care is possible?

Regarding prognosis:

Assuming diagnosis and treatment are accurate, can individual comprehend and follow medication treatment regimen including proper dose to be taking, what time of day to take medication, and how to increase dosage when ordered? If individual is not capable, is another responsible individual available to oversee treatment? If not, would individual benefit from hospitalization until self-care is possible?

Was individual made aware of possible side effects and what to do if a side effect is experienced?

Does individual have a good working rapport with his or her physician?

Does individual know how often to see physician and is transportation available? Is individual diligent about keeping appointments?

Has the physician informed individual as to what to do to improve response to treatment and which activities to avoid to increase the likelihood of improvement? Is individual engaged in psychotherapy?

What other support is available to individual? Family? Friends? Church? Support group?

- **Medical Codes**

ICD-9-CM:	296.2, 296.20, 296.21, 296.22, 296.23, 296.24, 296.25, 296.26, 296.3, 296.30, 296.31, 296.32, 296.33, 296.34, 296.35, 296.36, 296.5, 311
ICD-10:	F31.3, F31.4, F31.5, F32.0, F32.1, F32.2, F32.8, F32.9, F33, F33.0, F33.1, F33.2, F33.3, F33.4, F33.8, F33.9

- **Cited References**

Frances, Allen, ed. *Diagnostic and Statistical Manual of Mental Disorders (DSM-IV-TR).* 4th ed. Washington, DC: American Psychiatric Association, 2000.

Appendix 4: AADEP Fellowship Gradation Scheme

AADEP Fellowship Revised Case Report Reviewer's Analysis

Case Report #		
Reviewer:	Date:	Deadline:
If Category does not apply, a minimum of two (2) points should be assigned.		
Content Item		**Points Assigned**
I. Overall Length, Structure and Readability of Report (20 points)		
A. Length - adequate description overall (0–4)		
B. Structure (6 points)		
1. Report divided into labeled sections (0–2)		
2. Identifying information [biographical, referral source, purpose] (0–1)		
3. Short paragraphs - one topic per paragraph (0–1)		
4. Answers to critical questions clearly identifiable (0–2)		
C Well written / discussion clear to non-physician reader (choose one – 0–10)		
1. Well written / no confusion (10) or		
2. Some difficulty in following text (5) or		
3. Poor or confusing (0)		
II. Medical content - History and Physical Examination (34 points)		
A. Purpose of exam, with disclaimer (0–1)		
B. Date of Injury and Jurisdiction [P.I., W.C., etc.] (0–1)		
C. Examinee's employer/job description provided (if relevant) (0–1)		
D. Chief complaint stated clearly (0–1)		
E. History of injury/event elicited from Examinee (0–2)		
F. Past medical and surgical history elicited (0–4)		
G. Discussion of prior claims (if applicable) (0–2)		
H. Review of systems (0–2)		
I. Medications described (including if taken day of examination) (0–2)		
J. Social history, INCLUDING activities of daily living, hobbies, etc, both prior to and after claim, elicited and described in depth (0–4)		
K. Physical exam thorough/consistent with the Guide's Recommendations:		

1. Examinee's age, height, weight, sex, hand dominance included (0–2)	
2. Examination thorough and focused on area of chief complaint (0–6)	
3. Relevant ancillary areas also evaluated (0–2)	
4. Subjective versus objective "findings" differentiated (0–2)	
5. Use of distraction testing/Waddell's (if appropriate) (0–2)	
Case Report #	
III. Medical content - Diagnostic Testing and Record Review (12 points)	
A. Diagnostic tests ordered by Examiner stated, with interpretations (0–2)	
B. Diagnostic tests reviewed by Examiner listed and described (0–2)	
C. Medical records reviewed are listed and discussed	
1. Medical records listed (0–2)	
2. Content of records specifically described, separate from history (0–4)	
3. Potentially useful but unavailable records described and requested (0–2)	
IV. Impressions/Conclusions (34 points)	
A. Content	
1. Diagnosis specifically stated (0–2)	
2. Symptom magnification or not (0–2)	
3. Causation of diagnoses discussed in context of claim (0–4)	
4. Apportionment to old injuries discussed (0–2)	
5. Is Examinee at MMI or not? (0–2)	
6a. If at MMI, Impairment rating (if applicable) or prognosis given	
OR [0–2 for (a) OR (b)]	
6b. If not at MMI, need for further testing or procedures defined?	
7. Impairment rating (if applicable) performed correctly (0–4)	
8. Work ability/restrictions defined as permanent or temporary? (0–2)	
9. Physical capacities described [based upon objective findings] (0–4)	
B. Conclusions fit with history, exam, testing, records (choose one - 10 points)	
1. Conclusions fit (10) or	
2. Questionable fit (5) or	
3. Conclusions not justified/no fit (0)	
Total Points Awarded	0
Percentage of Total Points Possible (N/100) =	0.00%
Fellow Criteria Points (Percentage × 40) =	0
Reviewer's Comments: PLEASE PUT CONSTRUCTIVE, CONCISE, CRITICISM THAT THE EXAMINEE CAN UTILIZE EASILY	
Signature of Reviewer: MD or DO, FAADEP	

Bibliography

1. Babitsky S, Magravati J. Writing and defending your expert report. Falmouth: Seak, Inc.; 2002.
2. Martin D. Report writing. Proceedings of the Comprehensive Training Course, Chicago, Illinois, 1 May 2016. Chicago: American Academy of Disability Evaluating Physicians.
3. Brigham C. Independent medical examination report standards. Guides Newsletter; Nov/Dec 2002.
4. Demeter S, Washington R. The impairment-oriented evaluation and report. In: Demeter S, Andersson G, editors. Disability evaluation. 2nd ed. Mosby: St. Louis; 2003. p. 111–23.
5. Freeman G. Tips for writing reports. Conference proceedings of the AADEP Comprehensive Training Course, Chicago; 31 March 1998. Chicago: American Academy of Disability Evaluating Physicians.
6. AADEP fellowship case revised case report reviewer's analysis. Chicago: American Academy of Disability Evaluating Physicians; 2015.

Wacky Things That Happen After the Report Is Done and How to Deal with Them

10

Unexpected things can occur after an IME is conducted. Since most IMEs are performed as one-time events, the problem is that these occurrences often happen after the IME report has been sent. Several scenarios can create a bit of angst or anxiety for the IME physician. In this chapter, we list some of the more common "wacky things" that may come up and recommendations on how to approach them.

Claims That I Hurt the Examinee

Rarely will the IME physician be accused of injuring the examinee; however, these claims do occur. As we have previously indicated, these claims are especially difficult from a legal perspective because of the lack of the doctor-patient relationship within an IME. Thus, if the examinee is claiming that the IME physician injured them in some way, the process is usually pursued outside of the professional liability/malpractice process.

Injury claims are rare and usually unfounded because most IME physicians are very good at explaining at the outset of the process that there needs to be communication from the examinee if a physical examination technique is painful. Documenting within the IME report whether the examinee complained of increased pain or some other symptom within the context of the physical examination is therefore a good practice.

This is also an argument for using a post examination satisfaction survey or tool. Within the survey, one question that can be included is "Did you encounter any increase in pain during your IME?" Some IME physicians are more direct in their exit interview tools and ask directly, "Did you experience an injury during your evaluation?" If the examinee answered either or both of these questions in the negative, it is difficult to then try to show that an injury or worsening of the condition occurred simply as a result of the examination.

D.W. Martin, *Independent Medical Evaluation*,
https://doi.org/10.1007/978-3-319-71906-1_10

Claims That I Did Not Spend Enough Time

One the most common complaints if not the most common in the context of IME provision is that the physician did not spend enough time with the examinee. This complaint is often used by attorneys who are representing a party for which the IME report is unfavorable. Such accusations are made with a focus of attempting to show that the IME physician is not comprehensive with their history and physical examination.

First, there is some variability in the efficiencies of IME physicians in the history-taking and physical examination process. Secondly, there is no such thing as an accepted "normal" or "usual" amount of time it takes to take a history and conduct a physical for an IME. The reason is that the issues are variable; in some situations, the question may be only oriented to an issue of impairment rating determination, whereas in other cases, the IME physician may be asked to comment on several different injuries and comorbid conditions and determine impairments and activity recommendations for each or even more.

There are two practices that the IME physician should undertake to counter these claims. One is to make sure that the written report reflects the level of comprehensiveness that actually occurred with the history and physical examination. The other is to document the time actually spent within the report.

Documenting the time spent can be done is different ways. Some IME physicians elect to include a starting time and ending time for both the history and the physical examination. Others report the total amount of time spent in these two tasks. The report should also include the amount of time spent on reviewing medical and other records sent, as well as the time taken to review radiological studies. Lastly most IME physicians also document the time taken to generate the report. In this manner, the entire time spent on the work product (the IME) is properly documented so that there are no questions from any stakeholders involved.

Claims That I Was Not Thorough

These claims are also made by the examinee but are more often made by attorneys or other stakeholders in situations where the IME report is unfavorable to their client. Such claims are also sometimes made in the context of an argument where opinions of the IME physician are counter to those of the treating physician, and the argument is made that the treating physician must be correct because they have spent more total time with the examinee in the course of their treating relationship.

The focus upon the report reflecting the fact that the IME physician was thorough in their record review and history and physical examination again becomes critical. Just as we have indicated above, the report should reflect the level and time spent in the process.

When countering the argument that the treating physician opinion should be given weight over the IME physician's opinion, it is often the case that examinees will make comments about the approach and conversations I have had as the IME physician. Such statements that I have heard including "no one has ever spent this much time on my problem than you have," "you are the only doctor I have seen that has tried to understand what is going on with me," and "my treating doctor does not explain anything and at least you are asking questions" are actually quite common. When they arise, it is helpful to include them in the history portion of the report as it projects to the readers of the report the realities of the prior treatment interactions in a case.

There are also some literature studies that can be cited that have indicated that the IME physician evaluation is superior to that of the treating physician's. An excellent review of this subject is contained in the *AMA Guides Newsletter* article written by Barth and Brigham that indicates that treating physicians are best to avoid issues of forensic and legal questions concerning their own patients [1].

Phone Calls... "I Forgot to Tell the Doctor..."

There will be situations where the examinee has forgotten or wishes to include additional information that they want the IME physician to know about. Usually, the situation is such that despite the intentions of the IME physician in being thorough and asking several times whether there is any other information that is wanting to be addressed during the encounter, the examinee will call later in the day or even after the evaluation and want to clarify or add something. The prudent IME physician will include this information. The IME physician may delegate the collecting of this information to a staff member; however, the nature and general description of what the additional information is should be included within the history portion of the report and should be identified as to when it was collected and that it was conveyed via a phone call after the evaluations so as to properly record the chronology and events that occurred.

Occasionally, an examinee will bring in a diary or written information. These often are created from the examinee's perspective so that they are complete with their historical information. Some are lists that discuss symptoms as well as activities that the examinee claims they can no longer perform. Regardless of the information, the IME physician should ask if the examinee would allow the information to be copied. The copy can then be included in the report addendum. Most examinees would actually prefer that there information that they created be included in the IME report as many examinee's perspective is that their complaints have not been taken at face value. Acknowledging and even encouraging the inclusion of the examinee's own created document not only is a clever idea from the IME physician perspective but signals to the examinee that the IME desires to collect and analyze as much historical information as possible.

Additional Records Appear

There are many times that the complete medical record will not be available prior to the examination. The "extra" records often will appear a few days later or in some cases several weeks or months later.

An important job of the IME physician is to explore with the examinee that there is a complete record and understanding of all medical treatments that have occurred until the current time. During the course of the history taking, the IME physician will sometimes find out that there has been an evaluation or other treatment that has occurred that are not reflected within the medical documents provided. It is the IME physician's job to identify this in their report, and this often triggers an attempt by the requesting party to search for those records. Those records often then are sent to the IME physician for completeness, and in many situations the IME physician is asked to review them and submit and addendum to the report.

This is a perfectly acceptable practice, and the lack of a complete medical record being presented prior to the IME is a more common occurrence than what one might think. Of course, the records may or may not correlate with the history given by the examinee, and this is why it is critical for the IME physician to use the disclaimers at the end of their reports that were discussed in the report writing chapter so that the IME physician is provided latitude to change their opinion in these types of situations.

Letters from the Examinee's Attorney Arrive

There are many sharp and intelligent attorneys in practice. They will frequently try to take advantage of a novice IME physician or their staff. I continue to receive letters from attorneys (and other parties) that request a copy of my IME report because they attempt to treat that report just as any other medical record. Usually these requests are accompanied by the examinee's standard release for medical records that is HIPAA compliant. Do not fall for this. As was previously discussed, IME reports are usually attorney work products, and the standard practice is that the report can ONLY be released to the requesting party. If someone other than that is asking the IME physician for a copy, they should be referred to the requesting party as they are the one that should be asked, not the physician. It is obviously extremely IMPORTANT that the IME physician's staff understand this as well, and these requests are handled differently than the standard request for medical records.

Crafty attorneys will also send the IME physician letters that at first may sound as though they are trying to be helpful but which might have ulterior motives. Attorneys who are representing examinees who have upcoming IMEs scheduled by some other stakeholder may send the IME physician a letter that sounds pretty generic, might include some minor extra information, but then attempts to get information from the IME that they have no direct right to receive. An example of one such letter that I have received in the past is as follows:

Dear Dr. Doitright:

I represent Mrs. Alice King who is scheduled to undergo an IME at your office on May 23, 2017.

In addition to the medical records that you have already been provided, I wanted to let you know that Mrs. King recently was evaluated by Dr. Youba who has suggested additional surgery and to be off work indefinitely.

Once you complete your examination, would you be so kind as to send me a short note regarding your assessment of the need for this surgery?

Sincerely
Attorney Jerr Kuround

These kinds of letters seem pretty tame and innocuous; however, they are often veiled attempts to have the IME physician disclose information beyond the requesting party and should be identified and addressed. In these situations, I do not prefer to ignore them, but I will write the attorney back stating:

Dear Mr. Kuround:

I received your letter regarding your client Mrs. King.

As you know, IME reports are attorney work products and the reports are sent only to the requesting party. If you would like to receive a copy of my report on your client, you may contact the insurance carrier who requested the evaluation.

Thank you.

Sincerely
Dr. Aime Doitright

You Have a Complaint Lodged Against You by the Examinee to Your System or the Board of Medicine

These situations are frustrating but do occur. In 23 years of conducting IMEs, I have had two examinees contact my hospital vice president who is responsible for my clinic and lodge complaints against me in that they felt that I was an "uncaring" and "cold" physician. Both individuals filed complaints only after they received unwelcome legal decisions regarding their claims. Both happened to be within the workers compensation system. In one case, the examinee also completed a physician review on one of the more popular physician web-based rating sites and gave me one star out of five, indicating "don't ever go see Dr. Martin. He will write a bad report about you and use his brand of science against you."

At first, of course, I was upset. I wasn't quite sure what was meant by "his brand of science," but since I use evidence-based medicine and the scientific literature always to support my opinions, I eventually calmed down, and now these sorts of things don't bother me. I have long since understood that there are many "patients" who cease to be "patients" and turn into "claimants" because they are forced into a situation to prove their self-perceived issues as being legitimized. In these cases, I have found that it is rarely about medicine and the medical facts but more about feelings, motivation, and revenge.

I have also had two formal complaints lodged against me to the Iowa Board of Medicine. One complaint was that "He did not take care of my medical problem." That one was relatively easy to answer because all I had to do is show the Board of Medicine investigator the copy of the IME-informed consent that the examinee signed, which of course states that there is no doctor-patient relationship. The other complaint that was lodged stated "he only gives impairment ratings of 0% and never finds anything wrong with anyone." This was lodged by a claimant who complained of back pain and was seeking a several hundred thousand dollar permanent total disability award within workers compensation. The examinee had a normal MRI scan, an inconsistent history, many pain behaviors, but a treating physician who stated he could never work again. In this case I indeed did opine that his impairment rating was 0%, and the industrial commissioner hearing resulted in an award of $25,000, which is not atypical in my jurisdiction in these sorts of cases. In this situation, my communication to the Board of Medicine was to explain the role of the IME, to indicate to them that it is not I who makes the determination of his workers compensation award, and also then to provide several examples of IMEs where impairment ratings were given of something other than 0% and reports where there were more than ten diagnoses listed.

In each of these Board of Medicine cases, the complaints were dismissed. However, in Iowa, per statute, the complaints can never be expunged from the physician's record, so they will exist for eternity. If you think that is unfair, it probably is, but as is often stated, the arena of IME provision is a "contact sport," and if the IME physician is not prepared or unwilling to have to deal with these sorts of frivolous complaints, they probably should be doing something else.

You Receive a Subpoena Requesting ________ (Fill In the Blank)

As part of the IME process, you may receive a court order that demands that you do certain things. These things may be reasonable or unreasonable.

Certain subpoenas sort of make sense. If the court order demands that you send your report somewhere to someone other than the requesting party (often times a different stakeholder), that is not really a huge issue. Some court orders will require you to send your billing records on the case or ask that you send all correspondence in your possession. Those are also not "big deals."

There are other subpoenas that are really quite the opposite. Usually, these requests are made by attorneys who are simply interested in discrediting you or making your life disruptive. I have had requests to produce all of my IME reports that I have ever done in my lifetime. I rejected that request, as it would take my staff or me approximately 300 work hours to identify, copy, redact, and collate those reports. At one time, I wrote the attorney who had made that request about my professional time fees and that I would get started on that request right away as soon as I received a prepayment check for $100,000 for the amount of time it would have taken me to comply. That request went away.

My impression of these unreasonable requests are that the attorneys who make them are less interested in the science and medicine than they are to try to make your life difficult as an IME physician simply because your report is not favorable to their client. So what? Intellectual honesty and integrity mandates that the IME physician should neither be plaintiff nor defense biased. A frequent question comes up as to what is the ratio of "defense" v. "plaintiff" requests that I receive for IMEs. First, this is an impossible question, because I perform IMEs that originate from neither. Social Security Comprehensive Examinations are neither defense nor plaintiff oriented. I perform many IMEs at the request of the court system. But, the real answer that I give when asked is "I don't keep track because it is irrelevant. An IME physician is to be independent and unbiased. Thus, keeping track of whether an IME request comes from a defense or plaintiff perspective would by its very nature bias me from the get go. I am an advocate for the record and for the science of medicine. I could care less whether the 'plaintiff' or 'defense' side wins or loses. I have no dog in that show. "

Court orders also might involve demands for your personal financial records. Usually, an attorney is attempting to show that a large portion of your income may be coming from a source involved in the claim at hand. If you are an employed physician, this is less of an issue in that typically employed physicians are paid based upon a production formula that often will involve RVUs. Yet again, focusing upon the fact that the IME physician could care less where the referrals are coming from will pay dividends.

In any of these cases where subpoenas arrive, the IME physician should consult with an attorney. If employed by a system, the system usually will have counsel who handles these matters. In the case of an independent contractor or practice owner, the physician will likely have their own attorney. Many of these requests that are frivolous can and should be challenged, and even though it will take time and money to fight them, it will establish a principle where such requests can be avoided into the future.

You Are Deposed (and Sometimes the Gloves Come Off)

IME physicians should be prepared for depositions as the report is often a segue for such. Most depositions are pretty straightforward regarding the details of the medical issues at hand, but where the difficulties lie are usually in areas of disability. This book does not allow us to discuss in full detail the intricacies of attorney tactics of direct and cross-examination; however, the IME physician should prepare. My suggestions have always been to stick with what you know, don't answer things you don't know, and don't make things up. There is nothing wrong with an "I don't know" answer, but there can be all kinds of nasty things that can happen with a made up "on the fly" answer.

Some attorneys will try very hard to get under your skin, and some will even invoke what I call "attack mode." I have had attorneys question my religion, my political views, my education, and even my volunteer activities. What these have to do with the medical questions surrounding their client is a very good question, one that I have no answer for. Usually in depositions, I answer these questions with a preface of sorts, something along the lines of "I appreciate that you are interested in my views on (fill in the blank), and I am happy to discuss them with you, despite them being irrelevant to the medical and scientific issues of your client that I thought we were going to talk about today. If you think that our time today is better spent on talking about my (fill in the blank), then that is your prerogative, but it seems to me that since there are expenses involved with this deposition that you would want to focus on your client's medical issues."

You Are Designated as an Expert Witness and Are Scheduled to Testify at Trial

Every attorney will tell you that trials are expensive, and in most claims the focus is to try to settle the claim before it gets to court. However, there will be times when a trial occurs, and the IME physician may be called as an expert witness. There is no greater suggestion that I have than to BE PREPARED. Even if you are a rookie at testifying, or fear talking in front of people, if you are prepared and stick to what you have written in your report, things will be fine.

Again, this book is limited to the IME process, and there are other resources available to improve testifying skills if needed. The IME physician should be prepared to answer questions posed in trial directly, authoritatively, and at the same time appear professional and knowledgeable to the jury and judge. Answering the questions posed while looking at the jury instead of the attorney, wall, or ceiling will project credibility and improve communication with the jury as they will perceive a better connection. Also, slow down!! Physicians in general usually speak too fast, and when answering medical questions, one should not come away with the belief that the jury did not understand what you were saying.

You Encounter the Examinee in a Different Health-Care Context

There may be times when the examinee will return to a physician's office for some other issue. The IME physician will need to exercise judgment as to whether they can be involved with the care of a subsequent injury or illness but should not be involved if the new injury or illness has a relationship to the problems evaluated within the context of the IME.

For example, the physician should recuse themselves of determining fitness for duty in an occupational medicine setting if the issue surrounding fitness for duty involves a problem that was addressed in the IME. Opining on a permanent restriction regarding material handling because of a rotator cuff injury in an IME report would be seen as a conflict if the same physician is now being asked to determine fitness for duty if the job description required a certain level of lifting or carrying of objects using the shoulder.

Some of these situations may be more subtle. In situations where there may be a short supply of physicians to perform certain services, this may add additional angst in determining whether the IME physician can now fulfill a different role. In some cases, the timing of the IME in relationship to the current involvement can be important. Performing an IME 15 years ago in a case which has long since settled may not present as significant of an ethical challenge as one conducted just a year ago. In any case, each physician will need to determine what is practical and ethical for their situation, with the general guide being avoidance of conflict of interest.

Reference

1. Barth R, Brigham C. Who is in a better position to evaluate, the treating physician or the independent evaluator? Guides Newsletter; Sep/Oct 2005.

Bibliography

1. Husabo E, Monstad K, Holmås T, Oyeflaten I, Werner E, Maeland S. Protocol for the effect evaluation of independent medical evaluation after six months sick leave: a randomized controlled trial of independent medical evaluation versus treatment as usual in Norway. BMC Public Health. 2017;17(1):573.
2. Dell-Kuster S, Lauper S, Koehler J, Zwimpfer J, Altermatt B, Zwimpfer T, Zwimpfer L, Young J, Bucher HC, Nordmann AJ. Assessing work ability–a cross-sectional study of interrater agreement between disability claimants, treating physicians, and medical experts. Scand J Work Environ Health. 2014;40(5):493–501.
3. Spanjer J, Krol B, Popping R, Groothoff J, Brouwer S. Disability assessment interview: the role of detailed information on functioning in addition to medical history-taking. J Rehabil Med. 2009;41(4):267–72.

11 The Independent File Review

Independent file reviews are essentially independent medical evaluations without taking a history or performing an examination. File reviews are in most cases a bit narrower in scope that IMEs, focusing upon only one or two critical questions that the requesting party needs to know about.

Obviously, meticulously focusing upon the medical records presented becomes the focal point for the file reviewer. Establishing a trend regarding the care that is given from the time of diagnosis until the time of MMI or the current time is helpful.

File reviews are simpler when the questions posed are oriented toward asking about whether a treatment for a condition is reasonable and necessary or whether additional medical care is warranted. They are more difficult when questions are asked about causation or disability because the reviewer does not have the ability to ask their own questions which are commonly necessary to fill in gaps in the information that is provided in the record.

File reviewers cannot make determinations of impairment ratings based upon a record review alone. Although previous editions of the *AMA Guides to the Evaluation of Permanent Impairment* were not clear on the subject, the sixth edition of the *AMA Guides* now indicates that an impairment rating can only be authored after an appropriate history and physical examination is performed by the evaluating physician. There are times, however, when the file reviewer is asked to comment or critique an impairment rating given by another physician. This analysis is appropriate in so far as the file reviewer may make comments upon the validity of the impairment rating in so far as to whether the rating physician has followed the protocols and applied the criteria within the *AMA Guides* correctly. However, a specific impairment rating may not be determined because the file review is not able to conduct their own physical examination to corroborate the examination findings contained within the record.

As an example, let us consider a request for an independent file review where there is a question posed regarding the accuracy or validity of an impairment rating conducted using the *AMA Guides to the Evaluation of Permanent Impairment, Fifth Edition*, after a rotator cuff surgery. The range of motion values are recorded in the

D.W. Martin, *Independent Medical Evaluation*,
https://doi.org/10.1007/978-3-319-71906-1_11

records that are presented that were used to calculate the impairment rating and were applied to the range of motion tables regarding the shoulder that appear in the appropriate section of the upper extremity chapter of the *AMA Guides*. The impairment rating values that correlate with each of the six directions of motion measured of the injured shoulder were listed and added together, and an impairment rating of 6% of the upper extremity/4% of the whole person was determined. While the file reviewer is able to comment within their report about the appropriateness of the methodology of calculating the impairment rating in this case (it is done correctly according to the instructions), they would NOT be able to verify that the impairment rating is indeed 6% upper extremity/4% whole person because the file reviewer is unable to perform the physical examination and measure the range of motion using a goniometer themselves. There could easily be an error in the application of the goniometer (the range of motion was not conducted correctly under the *AMA Guides* instructions), or there could be validity issues with the range of motion values themselves. In either case, this could lead an independent medical examiner to a different conclusion regarding the absolute impairment rating number, but the independent file reviewer would be unable to know this otherwise.

With questions regarding causation, the file reviewer is often left to ponder whether the history recorded in file is accurate and often wishes that more detail exists. In many cases, there is insufficient information within the medical records to allow a file reviewer to determine causation "within a degree of reasonable medical certainty," and the file review report should explain what would be necessary in order to make a proper determination. In many file reviews where causation is in question, the medical records simply relate a time-related history of onset of symptoms, but lack any specificity regarding work tasks, or work injury details, thereby leaving the file reviewer in a quandary. Nevertheless, it is often best for the file reviewer to explain to the requesting party what the current medical literature on causation indicates would be necessary for the diagnosis in question to be deemed "caused" by work. For example, if a medical record has documented a carpal tunnel syndrome in a meatpacking worker who reported onset 3 months prior but no other details in the record exist, the file reviewer is best to explain within the report that they are unable to determine whether the work "caused" the carpal tunnel syndrome but that in order to associate carpal tunnel syndrome with the occupation, the occupation would need to be shown to include a combination of risk factors such as high force and awkward postures of the hand and wrist or high force and high repetition since this is what the medical causation literature indicates. If on the other hand the worker is an office worker who keyboards and no other information is given in the medical records, the file reviewer can state that keyboarding alone is not associated as an occupational risk factor for the development of carpal tunnel syndrome. (Note: both of these examples and occupational risk factor associations are contained within the *AMA Guides to the Evaluation of Disease and Injury Causation, Second Edition*, Chapter Nine, Carpal Tunnel Syndrome Section.)

Peer review or pre-certification reports are a type of independent file review where there is a specific request regarding the appropriateness of the medical care being provided to a claimant. Often times, there are questions regarding medications, injections, or surgical procedures that are being recommended. In these cases, it is often requested that the independent file reviewer have a discussion with the treating physician regarding the recommendation to obtain a better understanding of the rationale for the intervention. The file reviewer should approach this discussion with an open mind but at the same time understand what has been documented and what has not been documented within the medical record. The file reviewer should have a good understanding of evidence-based practice guidelines and what they state regarding the intervention in question. The file reviewer may ask the treating physician if they are aware of the EBM guideline perspective and delve into issues of why the recommendation is being made if it deviates from these guidelines. It should be noted that in some situations, the treating physician may not be aware of the medical guidelines and the issues, and this is an opportunity for the file reviewer to at least introduce them as a process of education. There are times, however, that a treating physician may be quite resistant to a peer review discussion and be angry that another physician (or a party who has hired them) is challenging their recommendations. Thus, independent file reviewers who must perform peer review discussions should have a bit of "thick skin" when it comes to these interactions.

Within the appendix to this chapter, examples of independent file review reports have been included, much the same as what was done regarding IME reports. Again, the names and specifics have been made up and do not relate to any real case or claim. They are included for the benefit of the reader so that they may see examples of how these reports are formatted.

Appendix 1: Independent File Review Report Examples

January 22, 2014

NANCY WILLIAMS
CLAIMS EXAMINER
RISK ADMINISTRATION SERVICES, INC.
P.O. BOX 89310
SIOUX FALLS, SD 57109-9310

RE: Elissa Battin
YOUR CLAIM#: 235287
DOI: 10/31/13
SS#: XXX-XX-5862
DOB: 6/11/1985

Dear Ms. Williams:

I am in receipt of your request, per your letter dated January 13, 2014 to conduct an Independent File Review, concerning the above named individual's claim of injury.

Thank you for your introductory letter that includes the questions that you need to have addressed.

You have enclosed the lady's South Dakota Employer's First Report of Injury, as well as relevant treatment records, which include those from the office of Wallace Fritz, M.D., as well as diagnostic test results.

ELISSA BATTIN
1/22/14
PAGE 2

Claim Summary

Ms. Elissa Battin is a 28-year-old female who works for Sanford Medical Center as a Registered Nurse in the Cath Lab.

This lady received an influenza vaccination that was administered to her left upper arm on October 31, 2013.

The day after this, she went to a massage therapist who noted a nodule in her left collar bone area.

She followed up with her primary care physician on November 5, 2013, and it was identified that this was a left supraclavicular lymph node. She subsequently underwent both ultrasound and CT scan imaging which noted 3 separate areas of lymphadenopathy. A fine needle biopsy was then performed on November 27, 2013 that returned lymphoproliferation compatible with a reactive lymph node change.

From a treatment standpoint, the lady has been advised simply to do conservative based cares.

Discussion

You have asked, in your letter, whether or not influenza vaccines can cause a reactive lymphadenopathy. The answer to this is that they can. While I appreciate your informal conversation with an Infectious Disease Specialist, I, frankly, do not understand the reasoning behind what he told you. All vaccinations work on the concept of creating an antigenic stimulus to the lymphatic system which, then, in turn, produces antibodies to said antigen. Obviously, the lymph structures must be involved in this process.

I conducted a literature search regarding this and would point to 2 articles that I identified.

The first one is entitled, "Lymphadenitis Caused by H1N1 Vaccination: Case Report," from *Vaccine* 2010 MAR 2; 28 (10): 2158–60. This is an article written by Toy, the primary author, that discussed an ultrasonography identified solitary lymph node that occurred in the supraclavicular area approximately 1 week after H1N1 vaccination. It discussed that there was a pathologic examination of this lymph node that did show evidence consistent with proliferative immunoblasts. The conclusion of the author was that lymphadenitis can be a side effect of H1N1 vaccination.

The second article entitled, "Axillary Lymph Node Accumulation on FDG-PET/CT After Influenza Vaccination," from *Ann Nucl Med* 2012 APR;26(3):248–52 is an article with Shirone as the primary author that talks about the accumulation of certain inflammatory markers in lymph nodes after any vaccination. This particular article does specify influenza vaccination and makes the point that ipsilateral axillary lymph node accumulations of this have been well documented.

It is, therefore, established in the medical literature that ipsilateral lymphadenopathy can develop after vaccination with influenza.

ELISSA BATTIN
1/22/14
PAGE 3

Specific Questions

In regard to the 3 questions that you pose in your letter, I respond as follows:

1. "Diagnosis and prognosis."

Answer: This lady has a left supraclavicular lymphadenitis. Her prognosis is good.

2. "Causation of the diagnosed condition to the influenza vaccine on October 31, 2013."

Answer: The left supraclavicular lymphadenitis was caused by the sequela of the influenza vaccine administered to the ipsilateral extremity on October 31, 2013.

3. "Can it be stated with a reasonable degree of medical certainty that Ms. Battin sustained an injury or trauma at Sanford that caused the diagnosed condition?"

Answer: I am not sure about the terms "injury" or "trauma." What this lady suffered was a left supraclavicular lymphadenitis/lymphadenopathy secondary to an unusual sequela from an influenza vaccination that was given in the ipsilateral extremity.

Conclusion

The above statements have been made with a reasonable degree of medical certainty/probability.

The opinions rendered in this case are the opinion of this reviewer. The review has been conducted without a medical examination of the individual reviewed. The review is based upon documents provided with the assumption that the material is true and correct. If more information becomes available at a later date, an additional service/report/reconsideration may be requested. Such information may or may not change the opinions rendered in this report. This report is a clinical assessment of documentation and the opinions are based on the information available. This opinion does not constitute, per se, recommendations for specific claims or administrative functions to be made or enforced.

If you have any questions with respect to this report, please contact me personally through the office.

Sincerely,

Douglas W. Martin, MD, FACOEM, FAADEP, FAAFP, CIME, CEDIR
Fellow, American College of Occupational & Environmental Medicine
Fellow, American Academy of Disability Evaluating Physicians
Fellow, American Academy of Family Physicians
Certified Independent Medical Examiner (ABIME)
Certified Evaluator of Disability & Impairment Rating (AADEP)
DWM/lap

October 21, 2016

DANIELLE DEFENCE
ATTORNEY-AT-LAW
FOOT HIGH WALL GROUP
2600 BIG AVENUE, SUITE 450
DES MOINES, IA 50000

RE: Smith v. Torch

Dear Ms. Defence:

Per your request, I have had an opportunity to review your submitted information regarding the above named action.

Thank you for supplying the voluminous amount of records and ancillary documents for my review electronically.

For a listing of the records reviewed in this case, I refer you to Appendix A attached to this report.

Case Summary

Amy Smith is a 53-year-old white female who has previously worked as a Certified Public Accountant. Ms. Smith began to develop symptomatology in 2006 consistent with a diagnosis of small fiber peripheral neuropathy. She filed a claim for long term disability with the Torch Insurance Company, which was initially denied and then subsequently, upon multiple appeals, was approved from a timeframe through and including 2013. After that point in time, a review of the medical and psychological data led Torch Insurance Company to terminate their long term disability coverage.

I have been asked to provide a comprehensive review of not only the medical information, but the other ancillary support information in this claim regarding the verifiability of the long term disability condition.

A review of the medical documentation indicates that this lady has previously dealt with morbid obesity, having undergone a gastric bypass procedure where she has lost a considerable amount of weight. The medical record would go on to indicate that, more recently, she has been diagnosed and treated for a fibromyalgia condition, as well as having been identified with Ehlers-Danlos Syndrome.

Based upon the current Occupational Medicine Specialty designation's determination of fitness for duty, which is based upon the risk/capacity/tolerance paradigm, this lady should have the capability to continue to work as a Certified Public Accountant on a full time basis without risk of harm to herself or others.

SMITH V. TORCH
10-21-16
PAGE 2

Discussion of Case

The medical record would document that Ms. Smith started to develop symptoms of dizziness with numbness and tingling in the extremities in 2006.

After presenting to her primary care physician with these symptoms, she was subsequently referred to physicians within the Medical College of Wisconsin. She was living in the Wisconsin area at the time. She had a variety of specialty evaluations and baseline diagnostic evaluations or tests conducted.

A Neurologist at that facility gave her the diagnosis of autonomic dysfunction, as well as autonomic neuropathy and postural orthostatic tachycardia syndrome.

A review of the medical records would suggest that there correctly has been some degree of concern about the specificity and validity of that diagnosis, from the standpoint of the various different tests and clinical presentations.

Indeed, autonomic neuropathies are typically either categorized as either inherited or acquired. The Medical College of Wisconsin physicians and, for that matter, a number of physicians, for a number of years after that time, assumed that this was an inherited or a genetic type of autonomic neuropathy. However, as one physician in the medical record has astutely indicated, there have been no genetic tests done that have confirmed this. Thus, my view is that it is more likely an autonomic problem that has no familial linkage.

Acquired autonomic neuropathies also are very difficult to delineate and to diagnosis; however, there are some characteristic features of the disease process. I would respectfully point out that, in this particular case, the objective basis for the issue is primarily due to a skin biopsy that identified a small fiber neuropathic problem. Indeed, if one looks at the medical texts and references regarding acquired autonomic neuropathies, one finds that there is a condition known as idiopathic distal small fiber neuropathy which has characteristic clinical features that are very similar to this lady's. It is more than likely that is the appropriate diagnosis to give this individual.

I can not necessarily assign, based upon the information that I have in the medical record, that a postural orthostatic tachycardia syndrome is a better diagnosis; or, for that matter, any other type of primary or secondary acquired autonomic neuropathy.

The most common acquired autonomic neuropathy is that from diabetes mellitus. One would naturally consider that as part of the differential diagnosis in this individual, given her significant problems with obesity. However, the medical record also does not seem to verify that is a concern.

As she has undergone a gastric bypass operation, it appears as though appropriate attention has been paid to folic acid and Vitamin B replacements, which also, often times, need to be considered within this differential.

SMITH V. TORCH
10-21-16
PAGE 3

The lady continued to report symptomatology secondary to these issues thereafter. She subsequently moved to Cedar Rapids, Iowa and established physician relationships in this area. She has had some other evaluations performed specific to her neurological issues. One of which was by a Dr. Talman, who is affiliated with the University of Iowa, who actually, in review of the entire medical situation regarding her neurological problems, questioned the validity of an autonomic abnormality.

A variety of physicians have been involved in review of this long term disability case and claim over time. There has been some variableness with regards to opinions concerning physical activity level.

There seems to be a preponderance of individuals who believe that this lady's physical activity is somewhat limited, but there have been differences of opinion as to whether or not it is sedentary, light or something different. There, obviously, are differences of opinion regarding her primary treating physician, Dr. Karen Harmon, who, no doubt, takes the position of a patient advocate, which would not necessarily be unexpected.

Regarding any issues with respect to mental health or psychological issues regarding this claim, the plaintiff and her representatives have indicated that it is their belief that her medical condition has led to some sort of deficiency, with respect to cognitive capabilities and performance. However, a careful review of the various psychiatric and neuropsychological batteries that have been administered to this lady over time, show that there are no deficiencies in those areas. Thus, the overwhelming thought processes by these evaluators has indicated that, at least from a performance standpoint, this lady does not have a psychological or cognitive barrier to functioning as a Certified Public Accountant.

With regards to the diagnosis of Ehlers-Danlos Syndrome, I would indicate that it appears that the medical documentation suggests that this was identified mainly as a result of genetic investigation. There does not appear to be a preponderance of symptomatology reflected in the medical record that is consistent with typical presentations of that disorder.

Regarding the more recent diagnosis of fibromyalgia, this has been subjected to evaluation both by local physicians, as well as a specialty physician and tender point injections have been done by Dr. Kim. Fibromyalgia is a common cause of chronic widespread musculoskeletal pain, often accompanied by fatigue, cognitive distribution, psychiatric symptoms, and multiple somatic symptoms. The etiology of the syndrome is unknown, and the pathophysiology is uncertain. Despite symptoms of soft tissue pain affecting the muscles, ligaments, and tendons, there is no evidence of tissue inflammation. Like other functional somatic syndromes, fibromyalgia has been a controversial condition. Patients look well, there are no obvious abnormalities on physical examination other than tenderness, and laboratory and radiological studies are normal. Thus, the role of organic illness had been questioned, and fibromyalgia was often considered to be psychogenic or psychosomatic.

SMITH V. TORCH
10-21-16
PAGE 4

Even more recently, there has been an issue with trigeminal neuralgia, which has been treated with injection therapy. Trigeminal neuralgia is characterized by recurrent brief episodes of unilateral electric shock-like pains, abrupt in onset and termination, in the distribution of one or more divisions of the fifth cranial (trigeminal) nerve that typically are triggered by innocuous stimuli. It is a rare condition that affects women more than men. Despite its low incidence, it is one of the more frequently seen neuralgias in the older adult population. The incidence increases gradually with age; most idiopathic cases been after age 50, although onset may occur in the second and third decades, or rarely, in children.

As one looks through the holistic perspectives of this claim and its implications, one is directed mainly to the issues of endurance, with respect to job tasks and job capabilities. The plaintiff states that she does not feel that she has the endurance or capabilities of doing the job as a Certified Public Accountant.

A CPA/CPA Consultant typically is identified as a position that is primarily of desk orientation. This does not require heavy lifting, which can accommodate either a sitting or a standing type of an environment, which requires a reasonable amount of writing capability, computer skills and communication skills.

The ancillary information that has been presented for my review includes not only video surveillance, but also a record of this lady's activities for volunteer organizations. It would appear that her involvement in these types of activities and what is included within the video surveillance does not show any degree of physical or mental limitations or barriers.

In applying the principles of analysis, from an occupational fitness for duty perspective, the general medical and scientific perspective that has been now formalized in multiple references indicates that it is, indeed, the case that physicians rarely, in the past, have concentrated upon the importance of the fitness for duty or return to work decision making process. It is important to understand that there has more recently been a focus on illnesses and injuries in situations that are non severe and for which there are many patients with similar problems who work, and yet, other patients who consult with physicians seeking medical information to support a disability application. As is the case here, and in those other cases that are similar, the disability phenomenon or construct is not obvious and both patients, employers and disability insurers request information from treating physicians and also from second opinion or independent medical physicians regarding their implications. In these cases where there is neither obvious severe disability, or obvious major pathology, similar to what we have here, there can be quite a difference of opinion. The question remains as to what weight should be given to the benefit of the patient regarding the return to work situation.

As a result of this, a more focused attention has been paid to what is commonly now known as the risk/capacity/tolerance paradigm. This paradigm is based upon the foundational principles that physicians can assess certain items of the equation,

SMITH V. TORCH
10-21-16
PAGE 5

but not all. As a rule, physicians are very good at identifying risk. They are reasonably good at identifying capacity. However, tolerance is not something that can be measured scientifically and it has been stated that tolerance is really not a concept or a subject that physicians can provide any type of opinion at all upon, given the fact that it is individualistic and is driven primarily by motivational issues of the individual patient.

More recently, this concept has been published by the American Medical Association in a textbook known as *The AMA Guides to the Evaluation of Work Ability and Return to Work, Second Edition.*

Applying this paradigm to this particular case, when one analyzes the medical record, it appears that there is insignificant risk for Ms. Smith to work as a full-time CPA/CPA Consultant (and certainly not in an intermittent part-time capacity). There does not appear to be any evidence of the medical documentation or ancillary documentation that would support a risk of harm to herself or others in that capacity. Thus, it does not appear that risk is an issue here.

It may be more appropriate to consider capacity, in that this is an area which takes into consideration the degree of strength, flexibility and endurance necessary in order to perform a particular job task. Although there appears to be some differences of opinion, with respect to this lady's capacity, most physicians have indicated, within their actual personal examination or review of the records, that this lady has some degree of capacity. Most physicians that have talked about this in the medical records that have been presented have used the dictionary of occupational titles terminology such as "sedentary" or "light." Although those titles often times are still utilized by practitioners, the current Occupational Medicine viewpoint is that labeling or categorization often times fails to yield the degree of specificity necessary to answer a particular question about a particular job. It is important to understand what the necessary physical demands are with respect to a Certified Public Accountant. As I have indicated previously, it is primarily a job that is frequently known as "sedentary," but rarely requires any type of strength, flexibility or maneuverability tasks. As it is a job that primarily is involved in mental task functions, the focus with regards to this particular disability claim should rightly be placed in those crosshairs. And, as such, given the objective information that has been communicated within the psychiatric, psychological and neuropsychological tests, there does not appear to be any limitation in that regard.

Therefore, the issue here primarily has to do with respect to tolerance. Tolerance is what is frequently known as a psychophysiological concept. It addresses the ability to tolerate sustained work or activity at a given level, and pays particular attention to reported symptomatology in that regard. Tolerance is, often times, stated to be dependent upon the rewards available for doing an activity that is in question. Frequently, when a patient describes his or her activity tolerances, a physician may

SMITH V. TORCH
10-21-16
PAGE 6

feel that this should be the basis for physician imposed activity restrictions. However, on a medical certification form, the term, 'work restrictions' means what the patient should not do on the basis of risk or harm to themselves or others. Symptoms alone do not harm. So, 'work restrictions' are not appropriate, if based only on symptoms.

This has led experts in the field to describe tolerance as not being a scientifically verifiable concept. This also explains why 2 physicians can have very different explanations and viewpoints with regards to concepts of work ability. When objective pathology is dramatic, physicians can generally agree upon what an individual should or should not be doing for work activity. But, it is less clear in situations for which there are not great degrees of objective pathology involved. This case is a classic example of that, in that we have objective information that is based primarily on a dermal biopsy that has shown an abnormality of a small fiber neuropathy. There does not appear to be any other objective basis that I can find within the medical documentation of verifying or validating other types of autonomic or other neurological concepts, save for an electrodiagnostic test that has shown a degree of carpal tunnel syndrome.

Therefore, the argument here is that physicians should not be involved in concepts or issues of tolerance, as that is an individual decision. The point of all of this description discussion is that tolerance has a lot to do with regards to motivational factors and the desire to perform and to also need work. It appears as though tolerance is the issue for the claimant, in this situation. Thus, from a scientific standpoint, it would certainly appear that this lady has little risk of returning to her full time job as a CPA/CPA Consultant, and has the capacity to do so. Therefore, from a medical and scientific standpoint, it is my opinion that this lady would have no limitations on her specific job tasks as a CPA/CPA Consultant.

She may have some job task limitations if she was doing some type of a job that required heavier physical exertion. I think that some of the physicians that have reviewed this lady's situation in the past have probably correctly identified some of those things. Although the identification of capacity, in this situation, is not well grounded because of lack of tests, such as a Functional Capacity Examination or other ability determinant analyses, it is probably more true than not that this lady could at least operate in what individuals have described as a "light" physical demand level. My general viewpoint on this is that this lady should, in general, be able to manipulate, from a material handling standpoint, 20 pounds. She should be able to sit, stand and walk with reasonable breaks. She may have issues with respect to balance, and I would caution her with regards to work at unprotected heights or situations where balance is important in an upright position, such as walking on uneven surfaces, standing on platforms, ladders and so forth.

SMITH V. TORCH
10-21-16
PAGE 7

Specific Question

I have been asked 2 questions in this case, which I respond to as follows:

1. "Does Ms. Smith have functional impairments from August 1, 2013 forward as a result of any 1 condition or combination of conditions? If so, please list the functional impairments and the evidence supporting your opinion."

Answer: I have taken into consideration Ms. Smith's situation with regards to the previously identified small fiber neuropathic abnormality identified on her dermal biopsy, as well as the previous labeling of an autonomic dysfunction or postural orthostatic issue. Also taking into consideration the fact of her previous morbid obesity, the fact that she has undergone a gastric bypass operation and has lost a considerable amount of weight, and the more recent implication of her Ehlers-Danlos Syndrome, her fibromyalgia, and other more chronic long-term medical issues.

It is my opinion that Ms. Smith probably does have some degree of functional impairment from August 1, 2013 forward, when one takes into consideration the combination or collaboration of all of these diseases and how they interplay into her activities of daily living. However, I think it is important to understand that these functional impairments, in my opinion, would not preclude her activity as a full time worker as a Certified Public Accountant.

In general, I believe that this lady would have the capability of material handling 20 pounds. I do believe that this lady would have some difficulty with respect to balance issues and I would preclude her from uneven surfaces, unprotected heights, ladders, platforms, etc. I think that she should be able to walk, sit and stand with reasonable breaks. I do not have any other rationale or basis to limit her in any other way, going forward.

In analyzing this issue, I did take into consideration the more recent diagnosis of fibromyalgia. One point about that medical condition is that all medical guidance documents and evidence based perspectives, including that of the American College of Rheumatology and the American Academy of Family Physicians indicate that, within that diagnosis, individuals should and must be encouraged and counseled to be "normal" with regards to both work and activities outside of work. People with this diagnosis typically are able to work full-time.

As I have indicated above, I do not feel that the Ehlers-Danlos Syndrome that has been more recently identified necessarily has manifested itself in the medical record with any degree of significant limitation.

As I have discussed, I think the small fiber neuropathic problem is likely idiopathic and I think that is the true diagnosis that exists.

SMITH V. TORCH
10-21-16
PAGE 8

As to how much it is implied with respect to any type of autonomic issue or hypotensive issue, there probably is some degree of that. However, I think to label this lady with a diagnosis of something other than that is not correct.

When we look at those issues primarily, and in combination with each other, there probably is some degree of functional impairment limitation which is based upon the small fiber neuropathic process. In this analysis, I have used my experience as a Disability Evaluator, as well as an Occupational Medicine Physician, but also, and even more importantly, in my experience as a Board Certified Family Medicine Physician. The reason that I say this is that, as I have indicated before, a small fiber neuropathic presentation often times is most common in individuals with diabetic neuropathy. As diabetic neuropathy is quite common, I think that one can use reasoned comparisons of other patients with diabetic neuropathic problems, as they often times will manifest themselves in the very symptoms to which Ms. Smith has. Utilizing that extensive degree of experience, I think bolsters my perspective that, while there is some limitation that likely exists in this situation, it should not be a limitation that rises to the level of being unable to be employed or completely disabled, from the standpoint of performing CPA/CPA Consultant functions.

2. "Please identify appropriate restrictions and/or limitations, i.e., sit, stand, walk, reach, carry, push pull, perform repetitive and fine motor hand activities, perform upper extremity activities on a full time basis, etc. based upon functional impairments you have noted above. Please, specifically identify specific documentation in support of your opinion that the restrictions are/are not medically necessary?"

Answer: Largely, I have addressed those issues in Question #1's answer above.

To reiterate, I think that this lady should be able to material handle 20 pounds. She should be able to walk and sit with reasonable breaks. She should be able to have unrestricted capabilities with respect to upper extremity use otherwise. I do not think that there should necessarily be any concern here about any other issues, vis-à-vis her occupational demands as a Certified Public Accountant.

The documentation that I have used in support of this analysis is the entire medical record, as well as the ancillary information that has been given to me. I think that, from an objective standpoint, what we have here is a verification of a small fiber neuropathy on a dermal biopsy. I think we have very little else in the medical record that can be specifically identified as an "objective" true record of any other issues. Largely, the reports in the medical records are of symptomatology. One also needs to look at the trend analysis, with respect to the number of years that this lady has been dealing with this condition. For example, I do not see in the physical

SMITH V. TORCH
10-21-16
PAGE 9

therapy records that there is identified any huge or tremendous issue with regards to any postural orthostasis abnormality.

The other information that has been given to me does not seem to support any type of cognitive or psychological dysfunction with respect to her job tasks.

This would also seem to be borne out, based upon the ancillary information that has been given to me, regarding her involvement in her volunteer activities, travel activities, as well as what is seen on the video surveillance.

I have noted that there seems to be some disagreement, in this case, regarding what the plaintiff's actual work as a CPA/CPA Consultant entailed. When you look at the financial records, it does not appear that her financial income was consistent with what an expected full-time CPA/CPA Consultant would necessarily make in a calendar year. Without knowledge as to why that might be, I do not think that necessarily has any implication here, with respect to my perspectives on this. I think that, because of the information related above, this lady should be able to work full-time in her occupation of a CPA/CPA Consultant. I think it is irrelevant whether the individual might work, for example, 50 to 60 hours in 1 week, and then perhaps have no hours for the next week. Since there does not appear to be any type of job task or requirement that requires a significant physical component to her issue, any type of claims of endurance or stamina would seem to be more oriented toward any claims of cognitive impairment. But, as I have indicated above, there does not seem to be any of that that has been documented in the information that I have been given.

I would conclude my answer to Question #2 by referencing the fact that there are consensus statements of many different physician organizations that talk about the importance of maintenance of employment or work as a part of an individual's better long-term outcome, from a health perspective. The consensus statements of the Canadian Medical Association, the American College of Occupational & Environmental Medicine, and the American Academy of Orthopedic Surgeons all recommend that physicians return patients to their usual work goals as soon as possible. They note that prolonged absence from one's normal roles, including absence from the work place, is detrimental to a person's medical, physical and social well-being. They go on to identify that withdrawal from normal social roles can occur when individuals are not in their work role, and can be destabilizing to the patient's mental, physical and social well-being.

More pointed studies, such as those that have been conducted by Waddell and Burton, indicate that individuals who are not working actually may have significant harm being done to them, such as a higher mortality rate, poor physical and mental health conditions, increased health care utilization, and other social negative determinants.

SMITH V. TORCH
10-21-16
PAGE 10

Conclusion

The above statements have been made with a reasonable degree of medical certainty/probability.

The opinions rendered in this case are the opinion of this reviewer. The review has been conducted without a medical examination of the individual reviewed. The review is based upon documents provided with the assumption that the material is true and correct. If more information becomes available at a later date, an additional service/report/reconsideration may be requested. Such information may or may not change the opinions rendered in this report. This report is a clinical assessment of documentation and the opinions are based on the information available. This opinion does not constitute, per se, recommendations for specific claims or administrative functions to be made or enforced.

Sincerely,

Douglas W. Martin, MD, FACOEM, FAADEP, FAAFP, CIME, CEDIR
Fellow, American College of Occupational & Environmental Medicine
Fellow, American Academy of Disability Evaluating Physicians
Fellow, American Academy of Family Physicians
Certified Independent Medical Examiner (ABIME)
Certified Evaluator of Disability & Impairment Rating (AADEP)
DWM/lap

References

AMA Guides to the Evaluation of Work Ability and Return to Work, Second Edition; copyright 2011, American Medical Association, Editors Talmage Melhorn and Hyman; published by the AMA Press; Chicago, Illinois

The Personal Physician's Role in Helping Patients with Medical Conditions Stay at Work or Return to Work; American College of Occupational and Environmental Medicine Position Statement; December 11, 2008

Preventing Needless Work Disability by Helping People Stay Employed; American College of Occupational and Environmental Medicine guidance document; June 27, 2006

The Physician's Role in Helping Patients Return to Work After an Injury/Illness; Canadian Medical Association; May 21, 2004

AAOS Position Statement on Early Return to Work Programs; American Academy of Orthopedic Surgeons; May 21, 2004

Barth, R.J., Roth, V.S., Health Benefits of Returning to Work: Review of the Literature; Occupational and Environmental Medicine Reports; 2003; 17:13–17

Appendix A

Records Reviewed
Amy Smith

1. Consultation and letters from consultation sources:
   - Alex Barboi, M.D.
   - Mark Burns, M.D.
   - Paul Darby, M.D.
   - Denise Davis, M.D.
   - Nick DeFilippis, PhD
   - Donald Feinsilver, M.D.
   - Karen Harmon, M.D.
   - Sunny Kim, M.D.
   - Donwook Lee, M.D.
   - Steven McIntire, M.D.
   - Sudhakar Misra, M.D.
   - Lucien Parrillo, M.D
   - Joseph Rea, M.D.
   - Kathleen Sawasky, M.D.
   - William Talman, M.D.
   - Randal Wojciehoski, D.P.M., D.O.
   - Mary Yellick, APNP
2. Listing of Prudential Insurance Company contracts relevant to this case
3. Expert reports:
   - Karen Harmon, M.D.
   - David F. Peterson, M.D.
   - Randal Wojciehoski, D.P.M., D.O.
4. Treating Provider records:
   - Laura Ledger, D.C.
   - Dr. Sedlacek of Anesthesiology
   - Dental records from Dr. Tyler Link & Barnes
   - Personal training records for Fitness Together
   - Dermatology records from Forefront Dermatology
   - Records from Gastroenterologists, P.C.
   - Records from Mercy Hospital and Clinics
   - Records from Neurology at the Physicians Clinic of Iowa
   - Physical therapy notes from the Rec Center
   - Notes from Steve Washler, LISW
   - University of Iowa reports, Dr. Genadry
   - Dr. Pryba
   - Dr. Kori-Graf
   - Froedtert Clinic and Hospital
   - Matthew Goldblatt, M.D.
   - Joe Barrash

CONTINUED

RECORDS REVIEWED, AMY SMITH (CONTINUED)

5. E-Mail correspondence documents and communications with the following health care providers:
   - Mary Yellick, APNP
   - Miscellaneous other notes regarding her treating physicians
6. Pharmaceutical records from OptumRX
7. Copies of a variety of health related text messages
8. E-mail correspondence regarding health issues
9. Records regarding Milwaukee County Contract Invoice and Support
10. Exercise tracking information
11. Additional listing of prescription medication correspondence
12. Correspondence regarding health club, fitness center and gym memberships and activities
13. Copies of photos of the plaintiff
14. Information regarding volunteer activities of the plaintiff
15. Correspondence regarding previous job activities of the plaintiff, including accounting manager, a position regarding duties and qualifications
16. Copies of requests and answers from both defense and plaintiff regarding interrogatory questions
17. Surveillance videos and surveillance reports from September 28, September 29 of 2010, as well as October 23 and October 26 of 2014
18. Copies of correspondence between Torch Insurance Company and either Ms. Smith or her attorney representatives
19. Deposition transcripts of the following:
   - Karen Harmon, M.D.
   - Randal Wojciehoski, D.P.M., D.O.
   - Said deposition of Amy Smith
   - Deposition of plaintiff's husband
20. Social Disability Case Analysis

Bibliography

1. Melhorn M, Talmage J, Ackerman W, Hyman M, editors. AMA guides to the evaluation of disease and injury causation. 2nd ed. Chicago: AMA Press; 2014.
2. Rondinelli R, editor. AMA guides to the evaluation of permanent impairment. 6th ed. Chicago: AMA Press; 2008.

Index

D. W. Martin, *Independent Medical Evaluation*,
https://doi.org/10.1007/978-3-319-71906-1

Made in United States
Troutdale, OR
07/01/2023

10916778R00143

Independent Medical Evaluation

Douglas W. Martin

Independent Medical Evaluation

A Practical Guide

Springer

Douglas W. Martin, MD
UnityPoint Health – St. Luke's Occupational Medicine
Sioux City
Iowa, USA

ISBN 978-3-319-71905-4 ISBN 978-3-319-71906-1 (eBook)
https://doi.org/10.1007/978-3-319-71906-1

Library of Congress Control Number: 2017963258

This Springer imprint is published by Springer Nature
The registered company is Springer International Publishing AG
The registered company address is: Gewerbestrasse 11, 6330 Cham, Switzerland

Foreword

Independent medical examinations (IMEs) are a part of the "expert witness" system in legal proceedings. Courts have long recognized that lay juries need assistance from "experts" to understand complex litigated issues in fields like engineering, medicine, etc. These medical evaluations by a non-treating physician are at times necessary for patients to have access to needed medical care or disability benefits and at times necessary for patients to have access to the court system.

Independent Medical Evaluation: A Practical Guide written by Douglas W. Martin, MD, is as stated a practical guide for any physician who is, or who wants to be, an independent medical evaluator.

The AMA Code of Medical Ethics (2016) discusses these evaluations (Sections 1.2.6 and 3.2.3). Similarly, individual medical (ACP) and surgical specialties (AAOS) discuss these evaluations in their statements of ethics.

Thus, independent medical examinations are an important part of the "practice" of medicine, and physician participation in these exams is needed by patients, by insurers, by governments, and by attorneys.

As this book points out, no medical school or medical residency trains doctors on how to perform evaluations for insurers, attorneys, or the court system or on how to testify. This is the void in education that this book has targeted.

The goals of this text are to interest physicians in doing these exams and to help those already doing them to do them ethically and well. While many sections of this text seem to be written for the physician who is not used to doing these exams, each chapter contains wisdom that will be appreciated by physicians with years of experience in this field. Most IMEs do not ultimately result in the physician testifying either live in court or by deposition, but if legal testimony is required after a deposition, the IME report is the outline for a physician's testimony, emphasizing the importance of writing the report well.

Thus, whether a physician is considering doing these exams or is already very experienced in this field, this book contains helpful philosophy and practical "how-to" advice. I recommend it to you.

James B. Talmage

Foreword

Independent medical examinations (IMEs) are a part of the "expert witness" system in legal proceedings. Courts have long recognized that lay juries need assistance from "experts" to understand complex litigated issues in fields like engineering, medicine, etc. These medical evaluations by a non-treating physician are at times necessary for patients to have access to needed medical care or disability benefits and at times necessary for patients to have access to the court system.

Independent Medical Evaluation: A Practical Guide written by Douglas W. Martin, MD, is as stated a practical guide for any physician who is, or who wants to be, an independent medical evaluator.

The AMA Code of Medical Ethics (2016) discusses these evaluations (Sections 1.2.6 and 3.2.3). Similarly, individual medical (ACP) and surgical specialties (AAOS) discuss these evaluations in their statements of ethics.

Thus, independent medical examinations are an important part of the "practice" of medicine, and physician participation in these exams is needed by patients, by insurers, by governments, and by attorneys.

As this book points out, no medical school or medical residency trains doctors on how to perform evaluations for insurers, attorneys, or the court system or on how to testify. This is the void in education that this book has targeted.

The goals of this text are to interest physicians in doing these exams and to help those already doing them to do them ethically and well. While many sections of this text seem to be written for the physician who is not used to doing these exams, each chapter contains wisdom that will be appreciated by physicians with years of experience in this field. Most IMEs do not ultimately result in the physician testifying either live in court or by deposition, but if legal testimony is required after a deposition, the IME report is the outline for a physician's testimony, emphasizing the importance of writing the report well.

Thus, whether a physician is considering doing these exams or is already very experienced in this field, this book contains helpful philosophy and practical "how-to" advice. I recommend it to you.

James B. Talmage